THE
EVERYTHING
THYROID DIET
BOOK

Dear Reader,

It is my pleasure to write *The Everything® Thyroid Diet Book*. As a registered/ licensed dietitian, nurse, and certified diabetes educator, I have had many patients with different types of thyroid disease. On a personal level, dealt with Hashimoto's disease for more than twenty years. In the past two years I have developed celiac disease. I also am dealing with the effects of sclero-derma morphea, which is another autoimmune disease that I have had for more than fifteen years. Many people with autoimmune diseases have more than one. I know, I have three.

I have many resources available to me because of my occupation, but still found it difficult at times to manage my diseases. As a very compliant patient, I have swung from hypothyroidism to hyperthyroidism as I was gaining control of my celiac disease, and my nutrition as well as my medi-cations were better absorbed. I now have gained control of my health and wish to share with you many of the things that I have learned.

Thyroid disease will always be a big part of my life. As I wrote this book, I learned many small facts for my own health. I hope you learn and enjoy this book. I wrote it for all of us!

Clara Schneider

MS, RD, RN, CDE, LDN

Welcome to the EVERYTHING® Series!

These handy, accessible books give you all you need to tackle a difficult project, gain a new hobby, comprehend a fascinating topic, prepare for an exam, or even brush up on something you learned back in school but have since forgotten.

You can choose to read an *Everything*® book from cover to cover or just pick out the information you want from our four useful boxes: e-questions, e-facts, e-alerts, and e-ssentials.

We give you everything you need to know on the subject, but throw in a lot of fun stuff along the way, too.

We now have more than 400 *Everything*® books in print, spanning such wide-ranging categories as weddings, pregnancy, cooking, music instruction, foreign language, crafts, pets, New Age, and so much more. When you're done reading them all, you can finally say you know *Everything*®!

QUESTION

Answers to
common questions

FACT

Important snippets
of information

ALERT

Urgent
warnings

ESSENTIAL

Quick
handy tips

PUBLISHER Karen Cooper

DIRECTOR OF ACQUISITIONS AND INNOVATION Paula Munier

MANAGING EDITOR, EVERYTHING® SERIES Lisa Laing

COPY CHIEF Casey Ebert

ASSISTANT PRODUCTION EDITOR Jacob Erickson

ACQUISITIONS EDITOR Lisa Laing

ASSOCIATE DEVELOPMENT EDITOR Hillary Thompson

EDITORIAL ASSISTANT Ross Weisman

EVERYTHING® SERIES COVER DESIGNER Erin Alexander

LAYOUT DESIGNERS Colleen Cunningham, Elisabeth Lariviere, Ashley Vierra, Denise Wallace

Visit the entire Everything® series at *www.everything.com*

THE
EVERYTHING®
THYROID DIET BOOK

Manage your metabolism and control your weight

Clara Schneider
MS, RD, RN, CDE, LDN

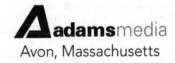

Avon, Massachusetts

An Everything® Series Book.
Everything® and everything.com® are registered trademarks of F+W Media, Inc.

Published by Adams Media, a division of F+W Media, Inc.
57 Littlefield Street, Avon, MA 02322 U.S.A.
www.adamsmedia.com

The Everything® Thyroid Diet Book contains material adapted and abridged from:
The Everything® Calorie Counting Cookbook by Paula Conway, copyright © 2007 by F+W Media, Inc., ISBN 10: 1-59869-416-2; ISBN 13: 978-1-59869-416-1.
The Everything® Diabetes Cookbook, 2nd Edition by Gretchen Scalpi, copyright © 2010 by F+W Media, Inc., ISBN 10: 1-44050-154-8; ISBN 13: 978-1-44050-154-8.
The Everything® Gluten-Free Cookbook by Nancy T. Maar and Nick Marx, copyright © 2005 by F+W Media, Inc., ISBN 10: 1-59337-394-5; ISBN 13: 978-1-59337-394-8.
The Everything® Guide to Being Vegetarian by Alexandra Greeley, copyright © 2009 by F+W Media, Inc., ISBN 10: 1-60550-051-5; ISBN 13: 978-1-60550-051-5.
The Everything® Guide to Macrobiotics by Julie S. Ong, copyright © 2010 by F+W Media, Inc., ISBN 10: 1-44050-371-0; ISBN 13: 978-1-44050-371-9.
The Everything® Low Cholesterol Cookbook by Linda Larsen, copyright © 2007 by F+W Media, Inc., ISBN 10: 1-59869-401-4; ISBN 13: 978-1-59869-401-7.
The Everything® Low-Salt Cookbook by Pamela Rice Hahn, copyright © 2004 by F+W Media, Inc., ISBN 10: 1-59337-044-X; ISBN 13: 978-1-59337-044-2.
The Everything® Soup Cookbook by B. J. Hanson and Jeanne Hanson, copyright © 2002 by F+W Media, Inc., ISBN 10: 1-58062-556-8; ISBN 13: 978-1-58062-556-2.
The Everything® Sugar-Free Cookbook by Nancy T. Maar, copyright © 2007 by F+W Media, Inc., ISBN 10: 1-59869-408-1; ISBN 13: 978-1-59869-408-6.
The Everything® Whole Grain, High Fiber Cookbook by Lynette Rohrer Shirk, copyright © 2008 by F+W Media, Inc., ISBN 10: 1-59869-507-X; ISBN 13: 978-1-59869-507-6.

ISBN 10: 1-4405-1097-0
ISBN 13: 978-1-4405-1097-7
eISBN 10: 1-4405-1155-1
eISBN 13: 978-1-4405-1155-4

Printed in the United States of America.

10 9 8 7 6 5 4 3 2 1

Library of Congress Cataloging-in-Publication Data
is available from the publisher.

The information in this book should not be used for diagnosing or treating any health problem. Not all diet and exercise plans suit everyone. You should always consult a trained medical professional before starting a diet, taking any form of medication, or embarking on any fitness or weight-training program. The author and publisher disclaim any liability arising directly or indirectly from the use of this book.

This publication is designed to provide accurate and authoritative information with regard to the subject matter covered. It is sold with the understanding that the publisher is not engaged in rendering legal, accounting, or other professional advice. If legal advice or other expert assistance is required, the services of a competent professional person should be sought.

—From a *Declaration of Principles* jointly adopted by a Committee of the American Bar Association and a Committee of Publishers and Associations

Many of the designations used by manufacturers and sellers to distinguish their products are claimed as trademarks. Where those designations appear in this book and Adams Media was aware of a trademark claim, the designations have been printed with initial capital letters.

This book is available at quantity discounts for bulk purchases.
For information, please call 1-800-289-0963.

Contents

Dedication

To all my readers with thyroid disease, I wish you health and happiness. In memory of my father Edward and my uncle Walter; they controlled their thyroid disease for many years.

Acknowledgments

Thank you to my husband Philip for his support in writing this book and as an active participant in my journey to better health.

To Amy, Eric, Lydia, Stephen, and Gia for their love and support in all I do.

I would also like to thank my endocrinologist, Dr. Giang Bach, for helping me with my rollercoaster ride with thyroid disease.

Introduction

IT IS AMAZING HOW many people have thyroid disease in the United States. The World Population Clock estimates the United States Population at more than 310 million as of October 2010, and approximately 27 million people suffer from thyroid disease. If you do the math, with these figures approximately one out of eleven people have thyroid disease. Thyroid disease is common in well-known people: Did you know that former President George Bush as well as his wife Barbara Bush have thyroid disease? Tipper Gore and Oprah Winfrey have it as well.

Thyroid disease in history is extremely interesting. Back in the mid-seventeenth-century, enlarged thyroids (goiters) were thought to be beautiful and a fashionable thing to have. In historical literature, surgery was done on them only when a patient had trouble breathing. Many people died from surgery at this time to remove the thyroid, and those that lived had problems with severe hypothyroidism. It was only 300 to 400 years ago that the thyroid was named by Thomas Wharton, and society today is fortunate indeed to have a better understanding of the thyroid and its functions.

A brilliant surgeon by the name of Theodor Kocher won the Nobel Prize in 1909 for his work in thyroid surgery. He developed a new technique for its removal and was strict with sterile technique. Later in his career, he lost fewer than 1 percent of his patients when he performed the operations. Hallmarks of his career also included gaining a better understanding of thyroid function.

In 1891, George R. Murray noted success treating a patient with severe hypothyroidism with sheep thyroid extract. In a little over 100 years, injections have been replaced by daily synthetic tablets for thyroid replacement. There is so much more to learn about how the thyroid functions and perhaps better ways to replace what is missing. According to diabetes literature, we are close to developing the artificial pancreas. In what year do you think we will be able to say the same thing about an artificial thyroid?

This book will help you understand your thyroid condition, whether it be hypothyroidism or hyperthyroidism. Options available for treatment in the year 2010 will also be discussed. If you have a chronic disease, proper nutrition will always help you stay healthy. Understanding a meal plan that stabilizes weight and offers healthy foods may be confusing. This is true especially if you have more than one medical condition that affects what you can eat. The recipes in this book have been analyzed for many different nutrients. You may not be interested in all of them. If you have a co-existing medical condition where this information is needed, then you'll be able to decide if the recipe can possibly be used. It should also be noted that the analysis of the recipes includes only the basic ingredients. If there are optional ingredients, you should account for them separately.

Reading *The Everything*® *Thyroid Diet Book* will answer many of your questions. Make sure all meal plans and medical therapies used are approved by your physician and medical team, including your dietitian, nurse, and pharmacist. Sometimes people have other members of their teams, such as a physical therapist to help with exercise. To locate a dietitian in your area, call the American Dietetic Association at 800-877-1600.

The meal plans in this book are just examples. The information provided is for you to get started improving your health and asking the right questions with your medical team. This book is not a replacement for medical advice. Ask your medical team what is correct for you, and don't be afraid to use the many resources at the end of the book. They should help you gain further understanding of the mighty thyroid!

CHAPTER 1

Thyroid Basics

If you or a loved one has a thyroid imbalance, it can be a frustrating drain on your overall health. You may feel constant fatigue, become depressed, feel irritable, or have serious trouble gaining or losing weight. Millions of Americans have thyroid issues, and proper diagnosis is the first step toward alleviating some of the problems you may face. But where should you start? Understanding the causes of your hypothyroidism or hyperthyroidism will help to form a plan to manage your symptoms and take control of your diet and health.

What and Where Is Your Thyroid?

The thyroid is an endocrine gland located in the front of your neck underneath your Adam's apple. It is very light and small—a normal thyroid usually weighs less than 1 ounce. It is usually compared to the shape of a butterfly. The wings are called lobes, and each lobe sits on the side of your windpipe or trachea. The middle of the butterfly (called the isthmus) connects the two lobes. Endocrine glands make hormones that are secreted into the bloodstream. Hormones are chemicals made in one part of the body that send messages to other parts of the body, regulating growth, metabolism, and mood. This is different from an exocrine gland, which secretes needed substances through a duct system—not through the bloodstream.

What Does Your Thyroid Do?

Your thyroid is responsible for making the hormones monoiodotyrosine (T1), diiodotyrosine (T2), triiodothyronine (T3), and thyroxine (T4). These hormones are made from tyrosine, which is a protein and the mineral iodine. T1 has one atom of iodine attached to the molecule, T2 has two atoms of iodine attached, T3 has three atoms of iodine attached, and T4 has four atoms of iodine attached. Your thyroid needs iodine to make these hormones. Iodine must be supplied by your diet, since there is no other way to acquire it.

FACT

T1 and T2 functions are less known and are rarely mentioned in thyroid health guides—T3 and T4 are typically classified as your thyroid hormones. In fact, most literature geared toward patients does not even mention these hormones. The scientific community needs to perform more research to learn the specific significance of T1 and T2 on your thyroid.

According to the National Institute of Diabetes and Digestive Diseases and Kidney Disease, thyroid hormones affect:

- Metabolism
- Breathing

- Heart and nervous-system functions
- Body temperature
- Muscle strength
- Skin dryness
- Menstrual cycles
- Weight
- Cholesterol levels

Thyroid hormones are particularly important in infants and children for proper growth and brain development.

If you do not have enough thyroid hormone, your metabolism will most likely be low, and there is a good chance you will have a problem controlling weight. Sometimes, people with too much thyroid hormone will lose weight unintentionally. Specialists do not endorse the use of thyroid hormones to lose weight, due to other undesired effects.

Calcitonin is another hormone made by your thyroid. It is made by parafollicluar cells (sometimes called C cells), which are different than the cells that make the other thyroid hormones. Calcitonin is thought to be involved in calcium metabolism. When blood calcium is high, receptors on the C cells stimulate the release of this hormone. Calcitonin that is made in the thyroid is called TCT, or thyroid calcitonin. It is thought that calcitonin is also made in other tissues of the body.

ALERT

If an individual has had her thyroid removed, calcitonin replacement is not given. Despite the amount of research on the thyroid, there has not been a thyroid calcitonin deficiency syndrome identified. It is thought by many endocrinologists and other physicians that when the thyroid is removed, the only thyroid hormone that needs to be replaced is T4, because the body can make T3 out of T4.

Testing calcitonin levels in the blood is not part of a routine screening for thyroid function, but your physician may test levels if medullary thyroid cancer or another disease of the C cells is suspected or needs to be ruled out. Five to 8 percent of thyroid cancers are of this type, and it is the third most common type of thyroid cancer. If this cancer is diagnosed, the treatment may involve removing the thyroid gland.

How Do Thyroid Hormones Work?

Your thyroid depends on your brain's almond-sized hypothalamus for adequate function. When your body needs more thyroid hormone, the hypothalamus releases a hormone called thyrotropin releasing hormone (TRH). This hormone goes to another part of your brain called the pituitary gland, which then releases thyroid stimulating hormone (TSH). TSH is released in the bloodstream and prompts the thyroid gland to release T3 and T4.

Think of the hypothalamus as the general store manager of the system, the pituitary as the supervisor of the system, and the thyroid gland as the stock boy who makes and stores T4. When the manager determines the body needs more thyroid hormone, she (the hypothalamus) sends out a message (TRH) to the supervisor (the pituitary gland) who, in turn, sends out his message (TSH) to the stock boy (thyroid) telling him to send out some T4. TSH is not the thyroid hormone itself; it is the message to the thyroid that the thyroid needs to release more thyroid hormone.

When your body needs less thyroid hormone, your hypothalamus releases a different hormone, called somatostatin. This hormone causes the pituitary gland to slow down the release of TSH.

QUESTION

What does it mean if my TSH is high?
The higher the TSH, the more thyroid hormone the thyroid is being asked to release by the pituitary. Sometimes the thyroid is able to make more and sometimes the thyroid cannot keep up. When the thyroid cannot keep up, you may be diagnosed with hypothyroidism.

Approximately 80–90 percent of your thyroid hormone is in two forms of the thyroid hormone T4. One type is attached to a protein called thyroglobulin, which is the storage form; the second is an active form, called free T4. When the hormone is attached to a protein, it cannot enter a cell for use. The more active form of thyroid hormone for metabolism is T3. T3 also has a form attached to a protein and free T3. Remember, T3 can be made from T4, so when a person needs thyroid hormone replacement, the form that is most often given is a synthetic form of T4.

Normal Thyroid Function and Diet

Thyroid function depends on the proper foods in your diet. Thyroid hormone is made from iodine and protein. Iodine is found in the soil by the sea, in animals that graze the land by the sea, and in saltwater fish and plants. It is also found in iodized salt, dairy products, and dough conditioners in baked products made in the United States. Iodine deficiency can lead to thyroid goiters, cretinism, and myxedema.

ESSENTIAL

Kelp, seaweed, and saltwater fish such as cod, sea bass, haddock, and perch are naturally high in iodine. Meat, fish, eggs, milk, and beans are high in protein.

A goiter is an abnormal enlargement of the thyroid gland that, over time, leads to the appearance of a swollen neck. A person with a goiter may have problems with swallowing, coughing, and sometimes breathing, especially at night. One of the reasons a goiter forms is a lack of iodine in the diet.

History and Research

Up until the early 1900s, an area of the United States was known as the goiter belt. The area affected included parts of New York State, the land surrounding the Great Lakes, and across to the Rocky Mountains. During World War I, men had a draft exemption if they had a large or toxic goiter.

One of the examining physicians for the state of Michigan was Dr. Simon Levin. Levin kept statistics on the problem and found approximately 30 percent of the men he examined had a goiter. Worried about the large proportion of men that could not serve in the United States Army, he was concerned about the public health implications for the citizens of his state and felt they could not be ignored. In a follow-up study in the Upper Peninsula of Michigan, he found approximately 64 percent of the population suffered from a goiter. Levin's work was followed by a study by R. M. Olen, the commissioner of the State Department of Health, in which out of approximately 32,000 school children in Michigan, 47 percent had a goiter.

Research was also taking place about this time in Ohio. In 1916, David Marine, MD, was given permission to conduct large-scale trials on school children in the state of Ohio. Children whose parents consented to treatment with iodized salt were the study subjects, and children whose parents did not consent were the control subjects. The results were amazing for decreasing goiters in the study subjects. Over 25 percent of the control group had goiters at the end of the experiment period, compared to 0.2 percent of the treatment group.

FACT

The World Health Organization (WHO) made a statement in 2010: "Iodine deficiency is the world's most prevalent, yet easily preventable cause of brain damage." The WHO is providing technical guidance around the world to aid nations with national iodization programs. The WHO has stated that when iodine deficiency is eliminated, it will rank with the elimination of smallpox and polio.

In 1922, Dr. David Murray Cowie, MD, at the Michigan State Medical Society recommended adding a trace amount of iodine to table salt in order to cure goiter. This idea originally came from Switzerland, where they added a small amount of iodine to table salt. Everyone uses table salt daily—this was Dr. Cowie's argument for iodine to be added. Dr. Cowie gained the support of the medical society for the addition of iodine to salt, and with their help they provided education to the citizens of Michigan. The society also researched the problems of mass-producing iodized salt. Dr. Marine was one of the physicians urging Dr. Cowie to ask salt manufacturers to mass-produce iodized salt.

In 1924, the Michigan medical society endorsed the use of iodized salt to prevent goiter. It was only a few months before iodized salt was for sale in grocery stores in Michigan. The iodized salt campaign was so successful in the state of Michigan that by 1932, 90–95 percent of the salt sold in Michigan was iodized. By 1946, one-third of the nation's salt was iodized.

Thyroid and Pregnancy

The American Thyroid Association believes that many pregnant women may be iodine deficient. They state that iodine is essential for the synthesis of thyroid hormones, and are worried America's iodine levels have decreased 50 percent in the past thirty years. Nonetheless, other than pregnant women, most Americans still get enough iodine in their diet.

ESSENTIAL

In the United States, commercial food manufacturers do not usually use iodized salt. During pregnancy and while breastfeeding, the American Thyroid Association recommends that women take 150 micrograms of iodine per day in a supplement, which can be included in their prenatal vitamins. They also recommend that food manufacturers use iodized salt, since Americans are encouraged to decrease their salt consumption and approximately 70 percent of the salt consumed is in commercial foods.

Cretinism is a form of mental retardation and stunted physical development that occurs due to a mother's lack of iodine during fetal development of her baby. In 1922 in a small iodine-deficient area of Switzerland, the sale of iodized salt was introduced. The results were amazing: Cases of newborn goiter disappeared. There were no new cases of infants born with cretinism, and the goiters in children were reduced in size or disappeared.

Required Iodine Levels

In adults without enough dietary iodine, a condition called myxedema may occur, causing hypothyroidism, because thyroid hormone can't be made. Symptoms of hypothyroidism include dry skin, body-tissue swelling, fluid around the lungs and heart, decreased metabolism, and a slowing of reflexes.

The last Recommended Dietary Allowance (RDA) values for iodine were set in 2001. RDAs are set to meet the needs of 98 percent of the population in the group. The Food and Nutrition Board of the Institute of Medicine of the National Academy of Sciences set the recommendations. Adequate intakes (AI) are provided for groups without RDAs. Tolerable upper intake levels are also provided. The units for iodine are given in micrograms (mcg) per day.

▼ RECOMMENDED DIETARY ALLOWANCES (RDAS) FOR IODINE

AGE	RDA OR AI FOR GROUP	TOLERABLE UPPER INTAKE LEVELS
0–6 months	110	Not provided
7–12 months	130	Not provided
Children 1–8 years	90	
Children 1–3 years		200
Children 4–8 years		300
Children 9–13 years	120	600
Teens and adults over 14 years	150	
Teens 14–18 years		900
Adults 19 years–70 years		1,100
Pregnancy	220	
While pregnant 14–18 years old		900
While pregnant 19–50 years old		1,100
Breastfeeding	290	
During lactation 14–18 years old		900
During lactation 19–50 years old		1,100

Excess iodine may induce hyperthyroidism, especially in some people treated for hyperthyroidism. This is one reason why there are tolerable upper intake levels of safety.

As you may assume, iodized salt is usually the main source of iodine for people in the United States. Saltwater fish and plant life are also good sources, as are plants that are grown in iodine-rich soil. Dairy products are also high in iodine. There are some medications that are high in iodine and erythrosine, which is red dye number #3, that also contribute to dietary iodine.

Other Important Minerals

A United States National Institute of Health Office of Dietary Supplements fact sheet advises that the element selenium may help prevent hypothyroidism. Deficiency of selenium may worsen the effects of iodine deficiency on the thyroid. If a person has iodine deficiency, he may also benefit from selenium supplements. As a caution, ask your physician if you should have a selenium supplement, as too much may be harmful.

QUESTION

Why are dairy products high in iodine?
The feed that dairy cows eat is high in iodine. Also, iodine is used to clean and disinfect the cow's teats at milking time, which introduces more iodine into the milk.

The Agency for Toxic Substances for the U.S. Department of Health and Human Services states in a Public Health Statement on selenium that it can build up in the liver, kidneys, blood, lungs, heart, and testes. Too much selenium can cause brittle hair, deformed nails, and loss of feeling in extremities. If large amounts are ingested in supplements, it could be life threatening. Foods that are grown in selenium-rich soil and animals that eat feed grown on rich soil have the most selenium values. In the United States, meats and breads are good sources of selenium. The Office of Dietary Supplements recommends eating Brazil nuts only occasionally because they are very high in selenium.

There are some limited studies that point to the need for adequate zinc and copper in the diet for proper thyroid function. Getting too much zinc appears to inhibit the absorption of copper. From a dietitian's standpoint, it would be prudent to have a well-balanced diet while achieving normal thyroid function. This would include eating a variety of foods and paying attention to any special needs you have. The soil that food is grown in will affect the amounts of nutrients in that food. It is therefore advisable to eat wholesome foods from a variety of places.

Signs and Symptoms of Hyperthyroidism

Hyperthyroidism occurs when there is too much thyroid hormone made in your body or if there is a problem with an overdose of thyroid medications. Your thyroid function has a lot to do with body metabolism, so if it is hyper, it tends to feel like your body is speeding up. Many of your body functions will work harder. This may happen very gradually, so the onset of hypertension may feel like anxiety or stress. You may not get all of the symptoms, but you could feel like a child that has had too much sugar, bouncing off the walls.

Signs and symptoms may include the following:

- Racing heart or heart palpitations and problems catching your breath
- Anxiety, nervousness, or increased feelings of irritation
- Tremors
- Trouble falling asleep or insomnia
- Excessive sweating; warm, moist skin; and intolerance to heat
- Problems with the digestive system, including increased number of bowel movements
- Physical or mental exhaustion and mood swings
- Increased hair loss
- Unexplained weight loss
- Enlarged neck area or goiter
- A change in the way that your eyes appear (bulging eyes or a stare)
- Loss of calcium from your bones
- Infrequent menstrual cycles and possibly a hard time getting pregnant

If you feel like you may have one or more of these symptoms, call your physician for help. If your doctor is considering a hyperthyroid diagnosis, simple blood work will most likely be done as a first step. Blood work for thyroid stimulating hormone (TSH) is usual. Remember that if you have a low or nonexistent TSH level, you most likely have *hyper*thyroid. TSH stimulates the thyroid to make more hormone, so if the TSH is low, there is no need for more thyroid hormone to be made. The American Association of Clinical Endocrinologists identifies optimal values for TSH at 0.3–3.0 mIU/L. Other blood work and tests may be done to confirm a diagnosis.

Your doctor may give you a manual neck exam—this does not hurt. You will be handed a cup of water and the doctor will feel your thyroid from behind as you swallow to help with a diagnosis.

ALERT

Make sure your doctor and medical team knows if you have a family history of thyroid disease. Also tell your blood relations if you have a problem. Thyroid disease tends to run in families, and you may be able to help one of your relatives and encourage her to call her doctor to get screened.

Signs and Symptoms of Hypothyroidism

Hypothyroidism occurs when there is too little thyroid hormone in your system. This can occur from lack of iodine or from the inability of the body to make thyroid hormone. It may occur due to congenital problems, surgery, or medications. It may also occur when there is a problem with the hypothalamus or pituitary gland. If you have trouble making thyroid hormone, the condition may take a long time before you feel any symptoms. In certain cases, the pituitary will send more TSH to the thyroid and your body may be able to keep up. Over time, the thyroid might not be able to keep up with the workload, and might not make thyroid hormone at the proper level. You might feel so tired that you want to curl up and sleep in any corner you can find.

The list that follows contains symptoms presented by the American Association of Clinical Endocrinologists for patients as thyroid function decreases. You may have all of them or only a few.

- Pervasive fatigue: A feeling of exhaustion that occurs even if you're sleeping more
- Drowsiness: Feeling abnormally sleepy during the day
- Forgetfulness
- Difficulty learning
- Dry, brittle hair and nails
- Dry, itchy skin
- Puffy face

- Constipation
- Sore muscles
- Weight gain and fluid retention
- Heavy and or irregular menstrual flow
- Increased frequency of miscarriages
- Increased sensitivity to many medications

If there is a problem with one or more of the symptoms that cannot be explained, just like with hyperthyroidism, call your physician for help. If your doctor is considering a hypothyroid diagnosis, simple blood work will most likely be the first step, as it is with hyperthyroidism.

Blood work for thyroid stimulating hormone (TSH) is usually ordered. Remember that if you have a high TSH level, you most likely have *hypothyroid*. TSH stimulates the thyroid to make more hormone, so if the TSH is high, the pituitary is sending a message to the thyroid to make more thyroid hormone. The American Association of Clinical Endocrinologists recommends optimal values for TSH at 0.3–3.0 mlU/L. Other blood work and tests may be done to confirm a diagnosis.

If you are diagnosed with hypothyroidism, keep in mind that it tends to run in families, so tell family members so they can also get tested. Older members of your family may have fewer symptoms of hypothyroidism and think their symptoms are simply due to just getting older or come with dementia; nonetheless, they may be thyroid related.

CHAPTER 2

Hyperthyroidism

Current statistics in the United States estimate that hyperthyroidism, the excessive production of thyroid hormone, affects as many as 2 percent of women and less than 1 percent of men. There are nine disorders that lead to hyperthyroidism, and it is caused by many different conditions. The symptoms of hyperthyroidism include those of a metabolism that is speeding up. A racing heart, nervousness, increased transit time through the gut (which causes an increase in bowel movements), trembling hands, weakness, and weight loss are some of the common symptoms that may be experienced.

Graves' Disease

Graves' disease, or diffuse toxic goiter, is the most common cause of hyperthyroidism in the United States. In fact, it is estimated as many as 60–80 percent of the cases of hyperthyroidism are due to this condition. There are approximately five times more women than men who develop Graves' disease. The condition is an autoimmune disease with a genetic component involved.

ALERT

Before having an RAIU, alert the physician of all medications you take, including over the counter herbs, vitamins, and minerals. Some medications may contain iodine, and substitutions may need to be made well in advance. Bring all medications to each visit for evaluation by your medical team. Discuss all allergic reactions, especially shrimp and shellfish allergies. Women need to discuss pregnancy and breastfeeding.

An autoimmune disease causes the body to release antibodies to attack and destroy the body's own tissue. In the case of Graves' disease, the antibodies stimulate the production of too much thyroid hormone. This process results in inflammation of the thyroid, causing hypermetabolism, which can include weight loss, trembling hands, increased number of bowel movements, nervousness, and rapid heart rate with palpitations. Over time, Graves' disease can lead to gradual loss of thyroid function.

If your doctor suspects that you may have Graves' disease, she may order tests to determine the following:

- Thyroid hormone levels
- Thyroid stimulating immunoglobins (TSI)
- Thyroid peroxidase antibody (TPO)
- Anti-TSH receptor antibody (thyroid antibodies)

Tests may also include a thorough neck examination. Radioactive iodine uptake (RAIU) testing may be ordered. This test is done in the radiology department of a hospital and measures the quantity of radioactive iodine absorbed by the thyroid, and also where in the thyroid the uptake takes place. If a great deal of radioactive iodine is absorbed evenly throughout the thyroid, Graves' disease is a likely diagnosis.

There are two conditions specific for Graves' disease that are not commonly seen in other thyroid conditions. The first is Graves' ophthalmopathy (exophthalmoses), which is sometimes called thyroid-associated orbitopathy (TAO) or Graves' eye disease. The second is Graves' dermatology, sometimes called pre-tibial myxedema.

Graves' Ophthalmopathy

Graves' ophthalmopathy is a condition where the eyes appear extremely large and seem to bulge out of their sockets. People with this condition have been known to have psychological issues due to the change in appearance. Many find this side effect more troublesome than the disease itself. Approximately one-fourth of people with Graves' disease suffer from this type of opthalmopathy. It results from an autoimmune reaction that causes inflammation to the tissue around the eyes. Often, Graves' opthalmopathy improves after one or two years of onset, but patients should visit an ophthalmologist regularly to prevent nerve damage to the eyes.

ESSENTIAL

It is important not to skip any doses of anti-thyroid medications. Your control of your thyroid disease may be compromised if you do. It is also important to take the medications at approximately the same time every day.

Graves' Dermatology

Grave' dermatology is less common in individuals with Graves' disease than Graves' opthalmopathy. Darkening of the lower legs and feet and fluid retention, or edema, are symptoms. The skin texture in the extremities may become hard, and has been compared to the skin of citrus fruit. The affected area becomes very itchy and bothersome. Identification and early treatment of Graves' disease results in a greater chance of this problem resolving, but sadly, the dermatology may develop even when the initial thyroid problems have been stabilized and treated. Topical medication to decrease inflammation and therapy, such as compression wraps, have been used in addition to thyroid treatment to offer relief.

Treatment

In the United States, the most common treatment for Graves' disease is the use of radioactive iodine to destroy the cells of the thyroid gland. As thyroid cells are destroyed, the pendulum swings, and a patient's condition switches from hyperthyroid to hypothyroid. When hypothyroidism develops, thyroid replacement will be needed for the rest of the person's life.

For a short period of time after treatment with radioactive iodine, the individual needs to be very careful around other people. The radiation given may cause discharge from the neck. The physician should be consulted about the length of time to be careful around others, and any special precautions that may be needed around pregnant women and children. Increasing fluid intake is often prescribed.

ALERT

In 2010, the United States Food and Drug Administration (FDA) added a warning to propylthiouracil label. This warning alerts consumers about reported severe liver injury and failure, some causing death in both adults and children. Patients need to be closely monitored when using this medication. It is not advised for children to use this medication unless they cannot tolerate methimazole, or if there are no other options.

Methimazole (tapazole or MMI) or propylthiouracil (PTU) may be used for mild Graves' disease. These medications may also be given to patients before other treatments, such as radioactive iodine or surgery. Studies have shown up to 40–60 percent of patients with mild Graves' disease may go into long-term remission, but years later may develop it again. The drugs need to be taken for up to two years for remission to happen.

Side effects of PTU may include painful joints, fever, stomach upset, itching, and a rash in less than 10 percent of users. A serious side effect of PTU is agranulocytosis, which is a serious decrease in white blood cell count. This occurs in approximately 0.25 people or 1 in 400 using the drug. Since white blood cells are needed to fight infection, any fever, sore throat, or other signs of infection should be reported to your medical team. Approximately 1 percent of patients who take PTU develop liver disease.

Another rare side effect of PTU is an inflammatory illnesses called vasculitis. This may happen even years after the drug has been discontinued. Isolated reports of congenital defects have been lower in patients taking PTU than methimazole. Surgery is used as a treatment for patients with Graves' disease who have problems breathing, potential cancer, or if the patient objects or cannot tolerate other therapies.

Toxic Nodular Goiter

The second most common cause of hyperthyroidism in the United States is toxic nodular goiter (TNG). With the increased metabolism levels of hyperthyroidism, there may be more heart complications as a side effect, as most patients seen with this condition are over the age of fifty to sixty years. As this condition occurs more in older people, they may not be able to handle the increased metabolism of the heart, and this may cause more heart complications. There appears to be a genetic component to TNG; it is not an autoimmune disease.

FACT

It is interesting to note that in areas of the world where there is widespread iodine deficiency, toxic nodular goiter is the most common cause of hyperthyroidism. In fact, in these regions, 58 percent of hyperthyroidism is due to TNG.

When a person has TNG, nodules in the thyroid develop that produce thyroid hormone independently of normal function. The result is excess thyroid hormone that leads to hyperthyroidism. The number of nodules that develop may vary from one to many. Patients with TNG typically have symptoms of hyperthyroidism, like weight loss, increased metabolism, sweating, nervousness, heart palpitations, exhaustion, and change in bowel frequency. If the nodules are large, they can press on the voice box or throat, adding potential breathing and swallowing problems. Nutrition may be compromised because of this difficulty. Changes in food consistency and texture may be helpful to aid in swallowing. Change in pitch and character of the voice as well as hoarseness may occur.

ALERT

If you have a goiter, you may experience problems with shortness of breath, depending on the position of your goiter. You may notice this when you're especially tired or when you move your arms over your head. Let your doctor know about this symptom.

Tests for TNG include a thyroid screening with blood tests and radioactive iodine uptake (RAIU) testing. With TNG, the RAIU will show the nodules or patchy spots where the radioactive iodine is seen.

As with Graves' disease, the most common treatment for TNG is radioactive iodine. Often, with treatment of radioactive iodine, patients with TNG will become hypothyroid. They will need to take thyroid replacement medication and remain under the watchful eye of a physician for the rest of their life. People with treated TNG may need to make lifestyle changes to control their weight.

Thyroid Adenoma

The National Institute of Diabetes and Digestive and Kidney Diseases (NIDDK) defines adenoma as a lump or nodule in the thyroid. Thyroid adenomas are common in the United States. It is estimated that approximately 5 percent of the population in the United States have nodules that can be felt. Many more people may have them, but they are so small they are not noticed by the individual or physician. Approximately 95 percent of adenomas are benign (noncancerous). It's important to see a physician if you think you have an adenoma so a proper diagnosis can be made.

The terms "hot" and "cold" are used when discussing thyroid adenomas. Hot refers to a nodule that produces thyroid hormone, and cold is one that does not. Many times physicians order blood work to measure thyroid stimulating hormone levels. Sometimes an adenoma may produce too much hormone. If there is only one adenoma, this may be referred to as toxic adenoma. Testing may include radioactive iodine testing, ultrasound, or a thyroid biopsy.

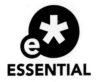

ESSENTIAL

The American Association of Clinical Endocrinologists recommends that everyone perform a self neck-check. To do this, you will need a mirror and a glass of water. Stand in front of the mirror and look at your thyroid. Your thyroid is located below your Adams apple in your neck. Take a sip of water and observe if there are bulges or lumps in the thyroid area as you swallow. If you see problems or have any questions, notify your physician.

Treatment for an adenoma is patient specific. If too much thyroid hormone is produced, an adenoma may be treated in the same way as toxic nodular goiter. In fact, the definition of having more than one nodule producing extra thyroid hormone is toxic multinodular goiter.

Thyroiditis

Thyroiditis is group of conditions caused by inflammation of the thyroid. Some of the conditions that cause inflammation lead to hypothyroidism and others lead to hyperthyroidism. One of the conditions that can lead to hyperthyroidism is postpartum thyroiditis.

De Quervain's Thyroiditis

Painful thyroiditis, also called De Quervain's thyroiditis or subacute granulomatous thyroiditis, is not an autoimmune disease, and is relatively rare. Usually, it is seen in patients that have had a cold or viral infection such as the mumps. This condition is difficult to diagnose, as the symptoms are the same as many other illnesses. Symptoms can include a very sore throat, jaw pain, or ear pain, and the thyroid can get very large. The pain can be on both sides of the neck or it may involve only one side. It is very important to go to the doctor, as some very urgent conditions may also have the same symptoms.

When the thyroid is inflamed, extra thyroid hormone may be released into the blood. If this happens, the blood work most often will be consistent with hyperthyroidism. Treatment may involve rest and medications that help with inflammation. Often, the condition will go back to normal over a few weeks to a few months. Sometimes the thyroid will not return to normal after an episode, and not enough thyroid hormone will be made. If this happens, you will need to take medication for hypothyroidism.

Postpartum Thyroiditis

Postpartum thyroiditis, or inflammation of the thyroid that leads to its damage, is seen in women up to one year following childbirth, miscarriage, or abortion. Up to 10 percent of pregnant women in the United States will develop this condition, but up to 25 percent of women that have positive thyroid antibodies (but display normal thyroid function in pregnancy) or type 1 diabetes will have postpartum thyroiditis. Women may feel tired, anxious, and emotional, or display other symptoms of hyperthyroidism that may be mistaken for typical feelings following childbirth.

ESSENTIAL

Make sure you and your loved ones are up to date on vaccinations to prevent viral infections. Cases of thyroiditis have been cited following measles, mumps, and influenza.

Typically, postpartum thyroiditis is not reported as painful. It usually develops during the first to sixth month following delivery. The following scenarios may happen:

- Inflammation causes the release of extra thyroid hormone and results in hyperthyroidism. When this happens, thyroid hormone production is decreased or may stop and the woman becomes hypothyroid. During this time, the woman will display symptoms of hypothyroidism.

The TSH level will increase and the thyroid function responds and returns to normal within a few months time.

- Some of the women will have significant damage to the thyroid from the inflammation and remain in the hypothyroid state. These women will need to take thyroid replacement.
- Other women have hypothyroidism that resolves without the onset of hypothyroidism.

Treatment of a woman with postpartum thyroiditis is individual and based on symptoms and her condition. Women with the condition have a greater likelihood of developing this problem again in subsequent pregnancies. They should alert their medical team that this is in their history so they can be properly monitored.

Acute or Infectious Thyroiditis

Acute thyroiditis is a type of inflammation most commonly brought on by a bacterial infection. Individuals with this type of thyroiditis often complain of neck and throat pain and fever. This is usually diagnosed by biopsy and blood tests. Once the source of the infection is determined, it is treated with appropriate medication.

Excessive Iodine Consumption

When large amounts of iodine are consumed, in most cases the body will increase thyroid hormone production initially and then decrease the amount of hormone produced so hyperthyroidism does not develop. Occasionally, when individuals with pre-existing thyroid disease consume large amounts of iodine, thyroid hormone production is blocked or reduced and hypothyroidism develops. This happens more frequently in individuals who have cystic fibrosis.

Some people with a pre-existing defect in the mechanism that shuts off thyroid production develop hyperthyroidism when an excess of iodine is available. This happens more in people who have lived in countries with little iodine available in the diet who move to a location where iodine is plentiful or they have a medical procedure that uses iodine-based contrast or medications that contain iodine. This condition is called the Jod-Basedow effect or phenomenon. On occasion, excessive amounts of iodine leads to painful swelling that will resolve when high levels of iodine are withdrawn.

Thyroid Cancer

According to the American Cancer Society, the diagnosis of thyroid cancer has been steadily increasing since the mid 1990s. It is the fastest-increasing cancer in the United States. However, even with the increase, the American Thyroid Association states that cancer of the thyroid is relatively rare.

The mention of the word "cancer" always evokes fear. This can be especially true with thyroid cancer because approximately 66 percent of the cases are diagnosed in people between the ages of twenty to fifty-five years old. When thyroid cancer is caught early and treated, the long-term prognosis is usually extremely good. In fact, statistics by the American Cancer Society show that the five-year survival rate approaches 100 percent for localized thyroid cancer of all types. Unfortunately, as the size of the tumor increases, and if the cancer spreads to the lymph nodes or travels to distant parts of the body, the survival rate decreases.

Most individuals with thyroid cancer do not have early symptoms. As the cancer grows, symptoms may develop. The National Cancer Institute recommends that a physician be consulted if you notice any of the following:

- A lump or nodule in the neck
- Trouble breathing or swallowing
- Hoarseness

It is not uncommon to develop a thyroid nodule as you get older, but they need to be evaluated by a physician to make sure they are not cancerous. Remember, diagnosis of thyroid cancer is based on a biopsy of a thyroid nodule or on routine screening of nodules removed during a surgical procedure. Statistics reveal that less than one in ten nodules contain cancer.

Cancer incidence in patients having thyroid surgery as a result of hyperthyroidism ranges from less than 1 percent to 9 percent. Pre-existing hyperthyroid conditions and the link with thyroid cancer have been studied, and results range between around 2 percent to up to 19 percent of patients. There may be an increased risk of thyroid cancer in patients with hyperthyroidism.

(Treatment of thyroid cancer usually includes surgical removal of the thyroid.) Partial removal may be discussed for some people, especially if they are young with small tumors. (Radioactive iodine therapy may follow surgery. With the destruction or elimination of the thyroid, hypothyroidism will develop and you will need to take thyroid replacement for the rest of your life.)

Overdose of Medications

All medications, both over the counter and prescription, need to be taken with care. Some medications, taken incorrectly, can lead to problems with hyperthyroidism and potential life-threatening consequences. It is important to discuss all medications and substances that are taken that may have interactions with the thyroid with your physician and pharmacist.

ESSENTIAL

If an overdose of medication is taken, MedlinePlus recommends calling a local emergency number like 911. The American Association of Poison Control Centers can also be called at 1-800-222-1222 twenty-four hours a day for emergencies or just questions. It is advisable to use a landline if possible, or if using a cell phone, make sure to let the educator know your location so they can properly route your call.

Medications that are used for the correction of hypothyroid conditions need to be taken as ordered. Brand names of many of the medications sold for hypothyroidism are as follows:

- **Levothyroxine (synthetic T4):** Levothroid®, Levoxyl®, Synthroid®, Unithroid®, and Levo-T®)
- **Liothyronine (synthetic T3):** Cytomel®
- **Liotrix (synthetic T3 and T4):** Thyrolar® and Euthroid®
- **Desiccated thyroid (which is made from porcine [pig] thyroid glands):** Armour Thyroid®

According to WebMD data from the American Association of Poison Control Centers' National Poison Data system, in 2008 there were 13,005 exposures to thyroid hormone preparations. More than one-third of the incidents involved children less than six years of age. Make sure all medication is out of reach of children to avoid potential problems. Peak serum levels when taking thyroid medications are within two to four hours for oral administration, and the onset of action for oral takes up to three to five days. Treatments to minimize absorption need to be administered within one to two hours of ingestion to have maximum benefit.

Overdose and reactions of medications that may cause a hyperthyroid condition may be related to taking more than the medication ordered by the doctor, or it could be from interactions with other medications. Make sure all doctors and pharmacists are aware of stopping or starting any medication, including anything over the counter. Some of the more common medications to ask about include:

- Diphenhydramine (Benadryl or other antihistamines): If this medication is taken, the dose should be determined by the physician.
- Iodine-containing medications, including contrast dyes, may cause hyperthyroidism in some patients that have been treated for Graves' disease or that have other thyroid problems. Iodine may also be in some expectorants.
- Some antidepressant medications may cause an increased therapeutic effect of thyroid medication. This may cause heart arrhythmias.
- Patients that need treatment with Interleukin-2 Therapy who have autoimmune thyroid antibodies may have problems with their thyroid during treatment.
- Patients taking levothyroxine that need to start indinavir may develop hyperthyroidism.

It is imperative to discuss how to decrease or discontinue every medication that is taken, with every member of the medical team. Care needs to be taken when discontinuing medications such as estrogens in birth control pills. Thyroid replacement may need to be increased when starting certain medications like birth control pills that contain estrogen. As patients discontinue these medications, there is a possibility that hyperthyroidism will develop. The physician that is in charge of thyroid status needs to be consulted for any change in all medications.

Ovarian Teratoma

According to the *Internet Journal of Surgery*, a very specialized form of ovarian teratoma called a struma ovaii is a tumor or neoplasm in an ovary that contains mature thyroid tissue as the predominant cell type. In 5–15 percent of cases, struma ovarii's will cause thyrotoxicosis (hyperthyroidism). Teratomas are often benign, but in rare cases can be malignant (cancerous). Presence of thyroglobulin, which is usually found in the thyroid, confirms the diagnosis of struma ovarii.

FACT

Struma ovarii are classified as monodermal teratomas. This means they are primarily composed of one kind of tissue. Other types of teratomas are classified as mature (dermoid cysts), which may contain more than one kind of tissue, and immature (malignant) teratomas.

Teratomas develop from totipotential germ cells, which are oocytes. Under normal conditions, oocytes will develop into an egg or ovum, but in this condition they develop into tumors that contain certain types of body tissues. Most cases of struma ovarii are seen in women between the ages of forty to sixty years old. Hyperthyroidism, acites, and pelvic mass are symptoms of this condition. Surgical removal of the stuma ovarii is usually recommended as treatment, due to the possibility of malignancy. Antithyroid drugs or radio-contrast therapy may be used before surgery to decrease thyroid hormone levels.

CHAPTER 3

Hypothyroidism

Many conditions can lead to hypothyroidism; it is extremely common in our world today. If statistics are correct, most of the readers of this book with a thyroid problem will have hypothyroidism. In fact it is estimated that in 2009, 10 million people in the United States had hypothyroidism. Symptoms of hypothyroidism reflect a slowing down of the metabolism. These may include extreme tiredness, problems losing weight, problems adjusting and tolerating cold temperatures, depression, constipation, decreased sex drive, and problems with memory and irritability.

Iodine Deficiency

The WHO has estimated that approximately 2 billion people are at risk of becoming iodine deficient throughout the world. This is about one-third of the world's entire population. Iodine deficiency is the leading cause of hypothyroidism in the world.

In the United States, the Food and Drug Administration conducts yearly total diet studies on amounts of nutrients that are in our food supply as part of the United States National Nutrition Monitoring System. These studies help monitor the safety of the food supply and determine if there are changes in vitamin or mineral status that may affect public health. More than 260 foods are analyzed for dietary iodine.

ESSENTIAL

Correction of iodine deficiency is normally based on adequate levels of dietary iodine. It is dangerous to take extremely high amounts of supplementary iodine. The advice from many health care professionals is to include foods that contain iodine in the diet such as iodized salt, milk, and seafood.

Demographic data from the National Health and Nutrition Examination Survey (NHANES) includes information on iodine status in the United States. According to the data compiled from 1988 to 1994, iodine status overall in the United States is sufficient. However, the consumption of iodine is falling, and more people in all age groups are considered iodine deficient. It is alarming to many doctors and scientists that 14.9 percent of women in their reproductive years are iodine deficient in the United States. This is particularly disturbing, as iodine is known to be essential to the developing fetus and in early infancy for brain and neurological function. The WHO recommends 150 mcg per day of iodine for adults, and if pregnant or lactating, 200 mcg per day.

Reasons for the decreasing dietary iodine in the United States are decreased use of iodized salt, reduced amounts of iodine in milk, and the reduced intake of cow's milk. Changing from iodized salt to sea salt decreases the amount of dietary iodine in the diet. Sea salt is low in iodine, with approximately 64 mcg of iodine in 2.2 pounds (1 kilogram). This compares to 400 mcgs in 1 teaspoon of iodized salt.

To evaluate iodine status in populations, urine levels of iodine are measured. The human body eliminates approximately 90 percent of ingested iodine. If very little iodine is excreted, it is an indicator of iodine deficiency. Evaluating levels of TSH, T4, and T3 is also used to diagnose low iodine status. If a goiter develops due to lack of iodine, a biopsy usually needs to be taken in order to make sure cancer is not present.

The synthesis of thyroid hormone is dependent on adequate supplies of iodine. Endemic goiters (goiter that develops from lack of iodine) may develop when iodine is missing from dietary sources or medication. For some people with thyroid disease, getting too little or too much iodine can lead to hypothyroidism. In normal thyroids, if there is excessive iodine, the body will block iodine from being incorporated into thyroid hormone. This prevents hyperthyroidism from developing. In some people, especially those with autoimmune thyroid diseases such as Hashimoto's or Graves' diseases, this mechanism does not work properly. If large amounts of iodine are consumed for a long period of time, hypothyroidism may develop.

FACT

In the late 1970s, results of studies conducted by the United States, titled "Food and Drug Administration, Total Diet Studies," showed a very high iodine level in many dairy products. The results were shared with the dairy industry, and the iodine-containing cleaning supplies (iodophors) were reduced.

Make sure you get enough iodine, but don't think that if a little is good a lot is better and excess is even better than that! In most instances, it's not a problem to enjoy foods that contain iodine. Ask your medical team for advice if you wish to start eating foods on a regular basis that contain large amounts of iodine like sea vegetables. Don't take excessive supplemental iodine (kelp tablets, large doses of iodine, etc.) without your physician's guidance.

Autoimmune Diseases

The function of the immune system is to protect the body from foreign substances that may attack it and potentially cause harm. Antibodies are made by the body to destroy these harmful substances. When you have an autoimmune disorder, your body makes antibodies to part of your body itself and it may destroy body tissues that are needed for normal function. Usually autoimmune diseases have a genetic component and need to have an environmental trigger. This section will address common autoimmune diseases that lead to hypothyroidism.

Hashimoto's Disease

Hashimoto's thyroiditis, also called chronic lymphocytic thyroiditis or autoimmune thyroiditis, is the most common cause of hypothyroidism in the United States and in areas of the world where iodine is considered sufficient. Two percent of the United States's population has been estimated to have Hashimoto's, with up to 10 percent of women over the age of fifty-five and 3 percent of men affected by subclinical hypothyroidism. Hashimoto's is less often seen in children. A person with subclinical hypothyroidism has elevated TSH levels, but T4 and T3 levels are normal. With full-blown Hashimoto's, there are circulating thyroid antibodies, a loss of thyroid follicular cells, diffuse lymphocytic infiltration of the thyroid, and the inability to make enough thyroid hormone. In some people, a goiter or noticeable swelling over the thyroid is also present.

QUESTION

Are there any genetic or environmental factors that will cause Hashimoto's?
According to the American Academy of Family Physicians, thyroid autoimmunity is inherited as a dominant trait. One may also need environmental triggers, such as excessive iodine consumption (the disease prevalence is in proportion to the intake of the population), radiation exposure from nuclear accidents, infection, stress, or pregnancy to develop Hashimoto's, but these triggers have not been shown to be conclusive.

Autoimmune diseases have characteristic symptoms of the body's own immune response, making antibodies that, over time, destroy its own tissue. In most cases of Hashimoto's thyroiditis, antibodies form that attack thyroid peroxidase (TPO) or thyroglobulin (Tg). Thyroid peroxidase is an enzyme in the thyroid that is involved in thyroid hormone production. Thyroglobulin is the protein that combines with iodine to make thyroid hormones.

If your doctor suspects Hashimoto's disease, she may order lab work to determine the presence of thyroglobulin antibody (TgAb) and thyroperoxidase antibody (TPOAb). Some people may have the antibodies without Hashimoto's disease. These people are at a higher risk of developing thyroid disease, so they should be periodically checked. Testing for TSH and T4 is needed to confirm the diagnosis of Hashimoto's and in order to select the correct therapy.

FACT

An antibody is a protein component of the immune system that circulates in the blood, recognizes foreign substances like bacteria and viruses, and neutralizes them. After exposure to a foreign substance, called an antigen, antibodies continue to circulate in the blood, providing protection against future exposures to that antigen.

Symptoms of Hashimoto's disease can be vague. During the stages of subclinical hypothyroidism, there most likely will be no symptoms at all. The body is able to keep up with making thyroid hormone, but the pituitary gland needs to send more TSH to the thyroid for this to happen. This is why TSH is elevated at this stage of the disease.

As time goes on, the thyroid is not able to produce enough T4, and classic symptoms of hypothyroid may develop. As patients feel the slowing of their metabolism, they may complain of fatigue, heavy menstrual bleeding in women, weight gain, and hair and nail changes. Hair may become thin and break easily, and skin may become very dry. Patients may also notice an increased sensitivity or intolerance to cold. As these symptoms may reflect other problems, patients may not report them to their physician. Women in childbearing years need to report a family history of thyroid problems to their physician and have their thyroid hormone levels checked.

Treatment of Hashimoto's consists of thyroid hormone replacement. Usually this is in the form of T4. Patients may be asked by their physicians to have periodic laboratory testing of TSH and T4 values. Over time, with progression of the disease, higher doses of replacement are likely.

ALERT

If Hashimoto's disease is not treated, complications may be severe. Goiter, heart disease, heart failure, osteoporosis, and depression may develop. In women of childbearing age, infertility, miscarriage, and birth defects may also occur. Myxedema coma is a rare but life-threatening problem. This medical emergency occurs when the slowing of metabolism leads to confusion and decreased blood pressure, heart rate, breathing, and blood sugar. The patient's lips and tongue may be swollen and they may have puffiness around the face. Emergency help is needed.

Ord's Disease

Atrophic thyroiditis or Ord's disease is not widely covered in the literature. It has been described historically as another type of autoimmune thyroiditis without goiter. Recent studies by Allan Carlé, MD, PhD, in the *Journal of Clinical Endocrinology and Metabolism* classify Ord's disease and Hashimoto's as extremes of the same disease with a normal distribution of thyroid volumes.

Postpartum Thyroiditis

Postpartum thyroiditis can develop into a form of Hashimoto's thyroiditis. Antiperoxidase antibodies are typical. Postpartum thyroiditis can follow three courses:

1. **Transient hyperthyroidism:** This is where the mother develops hyperthyroidism that resolves.
2. **Transient hypothyroidism:** Transient hypothyroidism follows transient hyperthyroidism. Hyperthyroidism develops, followed by hypothyroidism, and then the condition resolves.

3. **Hypothyroidism:** It is not unusual for women that have had hypothyroidism in the postpartum period progress with the disease process to full-blown hypothyroidism. In this case, the therapy would be the same as for Hashimoto's.

Thyroiditis

Thyroiditis is the inflammation of the thyroid. In many cases subacute granulomatous thyroiditis, or painful thyroiditis, starts out as an infection and thyroid hormone leaks from the gland to cause hyperthyroidism. This can be very painful. In many cases, the thyroid heals and normal function resumes. In other cases, the thyroid may be damaged, requiring thyroid replacement on an ongoing basis. Thyroiditis can potentially lead to hypothyroidism.

Reidel's thyroiditis can lead to permanent damage of the thyroid, causing hypothyroidism in approximately 30 percent of the cases. The inflamed thyroid becomes very fibrous and extends into adjoining structures. Medications used for this condition include steroids to reduce the inflammation. Tamoxifen has also been used to decrease the mass. Thyroid hormone replacement is needed if the inflammation causes hypothyroidism. If the trachea is compressed, surgery may be needed.

Surgical Treatments

According to the American Thyroid Association, there are many reasons thyroid surgery may be needed. Reasons include thyroid cancer, large goiters, noncancerous nodules, and overactive thyroid. The amount of thyroid that needs to be removed can vary from a very small amount (a biopsy) to the whole thyroid or a thyroidectomy.

Depending on why the surgery is done and how much thyroid gland is removed, a patient that has had thyroid surgery may not have the ability to make thyroid hormone. If this is needed and not replaced, hypothyroidism will develop.

Radiation Treatments

Treatments with radiation may potentially cause hypothyroidism, especially in children. According to the American Thyroid Association, during childhood the thyroid is much more sensitive to radiation than in adulthood. As children age, there are fewer problems with radiation treatment, causing hypothyroidism or thyroid cancer. As radiation doses increase in all age groups, the more likely these problems are to develop.

FACT

Discuss the different options available with your medical team if thyroid surgery is needed. The da Vinci thyroidectomy (sometimes called a robot option) may be possible. This surgery is minimally invasive; the surgeon has improved vision and access to the area. This type of surgery usually leaves no neck scars, and recovery time is usually faster than traditional surgery. Access areas are under the arm and a tiny opening in the middle of the chest.

Risks of radiation exposure include developing hypothyroidism. This may happen from a few months to a few years after exposure. Other problems that may happen include developing thyroid nodules or thyroid cancer. These problems may develop years after radiation therapy. If thyroid cancer develops, it is typically seen ten years after treatment with radiation.

Medical Treatments That Cause Hypothyroidism

Many medications may have an effect on the thyroid. The term "drug-induced hypothyroidism" refers to medication taken that causes a hypothyroid condition. Sometimes these drugs are taken to treat hyperthyroidism, and sometimes the drugs are taken for another condition.

Some common medications that are not taken specifically to reduce thyroid hormone levels may cause hypothyroidism. Lithium is used to treat bipolar disorder as well as other psychiatric conditions. Studies have reported between 5–20 percent of people who take lithium have subclinical hypothyroidism. In some people, lithium interferes with the production of thyroid hormone. Thyroid hormone levels are usually monitored, and appropriate therapy with thyroid replacement is typically ordered.

ALERT

Carry a list of all medications (and doses) to every physician and medical appointment. If any new medications are added, discuss potential side effects with the doctor and pharmacist. If there is a thyroid problem, discuss if the new medication may affect thyroid levels and how often thyroid levels should be monitored.

Other medications that can cause drug-induced hypothyroidism include:

- Amiodarone is a medication used for heart arrhythmias. This medication may have a side effect of hyperthyroidism or hypothyroidism.
- Steroid medication used to treat inflammation
- Sulfonylureas used in diabetes treatment
- Estrogen and birth control pills that contain estrogen

Many other drugs have effects on your thyroid. Some can cause drug-induced hypothyroidism, and some can cause drug-induced hyperthyroidism. Make sure the effects of all medications are understood. If there is an interaction that causes transient hypothyroidism, it is necessary to understand what to do when decreasing or stopping these medications.

CHAPTER 4

Hyperthyroid Dietary Concerns

Concerns about interactions between medication and food and nutrition are especially important to individuals battling an illness. With hyperthyroidism, weight loss can be an issue as well as weight gain. Many individuals with hyperthyroidism may need to follow a very strict low-iodine diet before certain procedures are done. Nutritional concerns such as dietary anemias and rapid turnover of nutrients such as calcium and vitamin D are also necessary to understand if you have hyperthyroidism. If you have hyperthyroidism, consuming a healthy diet is necessary for your well-being!

Medication Interactions and Food

Proper nutrition is essential for overall health, and if you have hyperthyroidism, your medication is essential as well. You need to be careful about making correct food choices concerning all medications. Many people have special concerns about a low-iodine diet. Others may have concerns if they have hyperthyroidism and diabetes and take medications such as beta blockers. Make sure all medications are disclosed to your physician, pharmacist, and dietitian so interactions can be discussed and you can consume the proper foods.

Possible Need for a Low-Iodine Diet

When testing for hyperthyroidism, a radioactive iodine uptake (RAIU) test may be ordered. If high amounts of iodine are consumed prior to the test, it will interfere with the results. You may be asked to follow a low-iodine diet for approximately two weeks before the test and sometimes for a few days after treatment. Ask the physician and/or medical team when to start and stop the diet and for any special instructions. Sometimes the laboratory where the procedure takes place also has special instructions.

ESSENTIAL

Ask the health care team if the *Low-Iodine Diet* published by the Thyroid Cancer Survivors' Association, Inc. is acceptable to follow for this time period. Copies of the diet and a special cookbook are available for no charge at *www.thyca.org/rai.htm#diet* or by calling toll free at 877-588-7904. Copies may be made for personal use or to give to a friend, but it is not allowed for publication in other books.

Beta blockers are sometimes used to help control some of the symptoms of hyperthyroidism, such as heart palpitations and nervousness, until the disease is controlled. Many people with hyperthyroidism also have diabetes. According to the American Heart Association, beta blockers may hide the warning signs of low blood sugar. This may happen because when this class of medications is taken, heart rate does not increase in response to a low blood sugar. In people with diabetes, careful monitoring of blood sugar is needed.

Possible Nutrition Concerns

There are many nutrition problems that may develop with hyperthyroidism, due to the hyper-metabolism and rapid turnover of body cells. Make sure symptoms such as fatigue are discussed with your medical team so you can test for certain conditions, such as the anemias. Getting help from a registered dietitian may be extremely helpful at this time!

FACT

Pernicious anemia is thought to be an autoimmune disease that causes a lack of intrinsic factor (IF) made in the stomach. Normally, vitamin B12 attaches to IF in the stomach and is carried to the last part of the small intestines, called the ileum, where it is absorbed. When vitamin B12 is not attached to IF, it cannot be absorbed and is excreted in the stool. A Shilling test can show if Vitamin B12 is absorbed by the body.

Anemia

Anemia is due to a decreased number of circulating red blood cells. When anemic, the body cannot carry sufficient oxygen to the cells, and you will be extremely tired. There are many reasons you could become anemic. Patients who have Graves' disease commonly have an anemia that resembles anemia of chronic disease. Anemia is diagnosed by taking blood work and measuring hemoglobin, hematocrit, and red blood cell count. After anti-thyroid medication has started, the anemia of Graves' disease will resolve in about 90 percent of individuals. If it does not, the physician may test for anemia related to nutritional causes. It is not unusual for patients to have iron-deficiency anemia or pernicious anemia, which is a deficiency of vitamin B12.

Vitamin B12 is found naturally in food that comes from animals (meat, fish, eggs, and dairy products). Cereals and multivitamins may be fortified with vitamin B12. One might incorrectly assume that by eating adequate amounts of foods that contain vitamin B12, pernicious anemia would resolve. This generally does not happen. The problem stems from lack of IF, so therapy usually consists of intramuscular vitamin B12 injections, or in some cases an intranasal (into the nose) form of vitamin B12 may be used. In severe cases, parenteral administration (infusion) may be needed. Untreated pernicious anemia can result in permanent nerve damage. Nerve damage can include weakness, numbness in extremities, and problems with balance. Approximately 5 percent of people with Graves' disease have pernicious anemia.

According to the National Heart, Lung, and Blood Institute, iron-deficiency anemia may result from blood loss, not enough iron in the diet, or the inability to absorb iron from the diet. Foods that are excellent sources of iron include red meats, oysters, seafood, and poultry. Nonmeat sources of iron contribute to iron status but are not as readily absorbed as meat sources. Nonmeat sources include cereals and grains that have been fortified with iron, lentils and beans, tofu, spinach, and raisins.

FACT

Foods high in vitamin C, such as citrus juice or tomatoes, will help iron absorption if consumed with the iron-containing food. Drinking tea and eating foods high in calcium will decrease absorption if ingested at the same time as the iron-containing food.

If iron is needed in supplemental form, blood should be drawn periodically to evaluate whether the supplements should be discontinued. The test for this is called a serum ferritin level. If iron is not able to be absorbed (usually due to problems in the stomach), iron injections and blood transfusions may be necessary.

Osteoporosis

Osteoporosis is a common complication of hyperthyroidism. According to the National Osteoporosis Foundation, it is a disease in which bones become fragile and more likely to break. All bones can be affected, but hip and spine fractures are especially problematic. When hyperthyroid, the number of bone remodeling cycles in the body increases, which can lead to bone loss. For proper bone health, adequate calcium and vitamin D need to be consumed.

Many physicians monitor vitamin D levels to determine if supplemental vitamin D is needed. A bone density test called a dual energy x-ray absorptiometry (DEXA) Scan helps diagnose osteoporosis.

QUESTION

What are good sources of vitamin D?
Vitamin D is considered the "sunshine vitamin," as it is produced from the ultraviolet light from the sun by the skin. Vitamin D is also obtained from dietary sources such as salmon, tuna, and mackerel. Other foods that contain vitamin D include specialty mushrooms that have been exposed to a controlled ultraviolet light while growing. Milk in the United States is generally fortified with vitamin D, but other dairy products are not. Look on the label to see if the product is fortified. Cheese and egg yolk have very small amounts of vitamin D.

Calcium is found in some food as well as in many antacid medications. If asked, most people will name dairy foods as containing calcium. Greens such as spinach, turnip greens, and kale also contribute to dietary calcium. Look on food labels for fortified sources, such as orange juice and other fruit juices, as well as soy and almond milk.

If possible, try to consume adequate calcium from dietary sources. The doctor or dietitian should advise how much each person should strive for daily.

Hyperthyroid and Weight

Hyperthyroidism causes an increase in the body metabolism, which can increase transit time of food in the intestines. Symptom of hyperthyroidism may include increased stool frequency, diarrhea, fatty stools, and malabsorption of food. Weight loss is a result of the problems that may develop. If a goiter is present, there may also be swallowing problems. Weight is lost in the form of body fat and also body muscle mass. As the hyperthyroid condition is controlled, a lower amount of calories and dietary protein may be needed.

ALERT

Doctors and dietitians sometimes recommend calcium carbonate and calcium citrate supplements for adequate dietary consumption. Ask your physician if this is recommended; recent studies have correlated calcium supplements to a 20–30 percent increase in heart attack risk.

Some people may gain weight when suffering from a hyperthyroid condition. This may happen due to increased appetite; thus, the individual eats a great deal more than needed. Weight gain is more common in younger people. In fact, in older individuals, the appetite may be decreased.

Suggestions for Weight Control

People with hyperthyroidism usually wish to know of a special diet they need to follow. Studies have not shown any special foods that have made hyperthyroidism better or worse, except for iodine. A balanced diet that provides needed calories is required for hyperthyroidism. Many times a heart-healthy diet is recommended. This includes eating fruits, vegetables, skim milk products, lean meats and fish, beans, and nuts. Consuming heart-healthy fats (olive and canola oils) and limiting dietary cholesterol, salt, and added sugars are also part of a heart-healthy diet.

A registered dietitian should be consulted for nutrition education of the hyperthyroid individual. Dietitians are trained to devise a meal plan that provides adequate nutrients and calories for patients. As nutrition needs change, they can alter the meal plans. They can also answer questions about new material that may be in the news or answer special questions pertaining to food and nutrition needs.

Weight gain after hyperthyroid treatment has been studied. It is not uncommon to gain up to twelve pounds in two years following treatment.

People with a history of obesity and who develop hypothyroidism following treatment are more likely to gain weight.

FACT

In 1984, there was a condition known as hamburger hyperthyroidism. It was caused by ingesting the bovine thyroid gland as part of ground beef. The outbreak resulted in the restriction of gullet trimmings in the products of cattle and pigs. Farmers and hunters who process their own meats need to be aware of this potential problem.

Staying Healthy with Hyperthyroidism

Many changes may occur in patients with hyperthyroidism. Make sure that open communication of problems and concerns exists with your health care team. Sometimes there is a change that one may not attribute to hyperthyroidism. These may include the following:

- An increase in thirst followed by an increase in urine frequency. Make sure the medical team is told, because you may also need to be tested for diabetes.
- Problems getting to sleep and waking before rested. Hidden sources of caffeine or stimulants can be discussed, as well as relaxation techniques and perhaps medication.
- Problems with concentration and attention. If it is caused by hyperthyroidism, this may improve with treatment.
- Sometimes in the elderly with Graves' disease, constipation is a problem. The medical team should be consulted. Advice needs to be given on how much fluid and fiber is needed per day as well as exercise recommendations. All health problems and concerns should be addressed to the health care team.
- Alert the medical team of all over-the-counter medications as well as vitamins and supplements consumed. There may be an interaction with your therapies or with the disease itself. Examples are kelp tablets or medications or supplements that contain iodine, which may possibly aggravate or cause hyperthyroidism in some people.

CHAPTER 5

Hypothyroid
Dietary Concerns

Individuals with hypothyroidism may have many dietary concerns. Goiterogenic properties of foods may be questioned. Many times weight gain is an issue. Other issues include possible constipation and issues that surround a decrease in metabolism. If this pertains to you or a loved one, read over every section in this chapter. What appears to be a very minor hint may lead to much more comfort and satisfaction in controlling hypothyroidism!

Medication Interactions and Food

According to a report published in 2001 jointly by the American Thyroid Association, the Endocrine Society, and Thyroid Cancer Survivors' Association, there were 13 million patients in the United States that took thyroid hormone (thyroxine or T4) replacement. One of the top selling brands of thyroxine is Synthroid (levothyroxine sodium tablets). When taking thyroxine, you need to be very careful with food-medication interactions in order to get the optimal absorption of this medication. On the manufacturer's website for Synthroid, the following guidelines are given:

1. Take this medication on an empty stomach. The recommendations are one half to one hour before breakfast. Synthroid absorption will be increased when the stomach is empty.
2. The following foods may bind to the medication and decrease the amount absorbed: soybean flour (infant formula), cotton seed meal, and walnuts. Dietary fiber may also decrease absorption.
3. Iron and calcium tablets as well as antacids need to be taken at least four hours before or four hours after taking Synthroid.

ALERT

MedlinePlus suggests taking levothyroxine tablets with a full glass of water. If this is not done, the tablet may cause choking and gagging or get stuck in your throat. This feeling is extremely uncomfortable!

The time that thyroid hormone is taken during the day has been the topic of various studies. A 2009 study by T. G. Bach-Huynh and colleagues in the *Journal of Clinical Endocrinology and Metabolism* showed that for one to get the most stable TSH level, thyroid hormone (levothyroxine) should be taken in a fasting state before breakfast as opposed to taking it with breakfast (at the meal) or at bedtime. This supports the recommendation from the manufacturers of Synthroid as discussed above.

Levothroid, which is a different brand of levothyroxine, contains lactose. If you have a problem with lactose intolerance, alert the physician because another brand may be recommended.

The use of thyroid hormones over time may speed up the process of bone remodeling. Over time, this may decrease bone density. A densitometry or DXA scan may be used to check bone status. Vitamin D levels may be checked by blood testing and monitored. Your physician may order supplementary vitamin D and calcium if needed.

Possible Nutrition Concerns

Changes in the way the body metabolizes carbohydrates and fats may take place if you have hypothyroidism. Remember, metabolism is decreased in the hypothyroid state. Carbohydrate metabolism is affected by decreasing the absorption rate of glucose (sugar). The ability of the body to break down the hormone insulin is decreased. In patients with diabetes, blood sugar should be monitored and insulin many need to be decreased as necessary because of this effect.

FACT

According to the American Thyroid Association, when hypothyroidism is treated, usually less than 10 percent of body weight is lost. A great portion of this weight loss is due to the excess water that was gained due to untreated hypothyroidism. Their opinion is that once the hypothyroidism is corrected, the ability to lose weight is the same as people without hypothyroidism.

There may be a change in serum lipids or fats with hypothyroidism. Serum cholesterol and low-density lipoprotein (LDL) cholesterol are often increased. Make sure to have these levels monitored as recommended by your medical team. The transit time in the gastrointestinal tract also slows. Constipation and distention may result as well. Due to the interference of fiber with thyroid hormone replacement, be careful not to consume fiber at the same time as your medications.

There are foods that are sometimes referred to as goiterogenic, or able to cause a goiter. These foods may block the uptake of iodine by the thyroid, leading to hypothyroidism. This may be a concern if iodine is marginal in the diet. Most people in the United States consume adequate iodine, so this is not a concern. Sulfur-containing cruciferous vegetables that are thought to help prevent cancer are actually part of this group. Examples are broccoli, cauliflower, cabbage, kale, and bok choy. Usually this is not a dietary concern recommended by health care professionals, but it does not hurt to ask to make sure there are no restrictions.

Soy products also contain goiterogenic properties if iodine is deficient. The National Institute of Environmental Health Sciences published a paper stating that in rats fed supplemental genistein, a component of soy, thyroid peroxidase decreased according to the dose. Thyroid peroxidase is the enzyme involved in synthesizing thyroid hormone in the thyroid. The researchers stated that high-quality human research needs to be done in this area. Other foods associated with goiters include millet, rutabagas, peaches, peas, strawberries, spinach, walnuts, and radishes.

QUESTION

What will decrease the tendencies of these foods to cause goiters? Studies have shown if these foods are shredded, it will decrease the compounds that cause goiter by 77 percent. If they are boiled, up to 95 percent of the compounds will be lost.

Goiterogenic foods are healthy in so many ways—they contain many vitamins and minerals and are an integral part of a healthy diet. Ask your health care team for specific individual recommendations.

Hypothyroid and Weight

Thyroid hormone is very important in the regulation of metabolism, which affects body weight. In individuals with hypothyroidism, basal metabolic rate is low. Basal metabolic rate is the amount of calories needed to stay alive in a resting state. A weight gain of approximately five to ten pounds is associated with hypothyroidism. Much of the weight gain is thought to be due to an increase in water and salt.

As a person on thyroid replacement loses weight, the amount of medication usually needs to be decreased. The medical team needs to be alerted to changes in weight so proper doses of medication can be ordered and you do not go into a hyperthyroid state. It is important to use thyroid medications as directed by your health care team. Drug manufacturers have issued warnings to not use them in the treatment of obesity or weight loss.

ALERT

"Thyroid hormones, including SYNTHROID, should not be used either alone or in combination with other medicines for the treatment of obesity or weight loss. In patients with normal thyroid levels, doses of SYNTHROID within the typical range used for hormone replacement are not effective for weight loss. Larger doses may result in serious or even life-threatening effects, especially when used in combination with certain other drugs used to reduce appetite." (Retrieved from the Synthroid website, October 3, 2010)

Suggestions for Weight Control

How much is known about weight control and our thyroid? As mentioned, when an individual has hypothyroidism, approximately five to ten pounds of weight can be attributed to the condition. Studies on weight control in hypothyroid patients have shown that a gastric (stomach) peptide called ghrelin is increased in the hypothyroid state. Ghrelin is sometimes known as the hunger hormone. Some studies have found it to be elevated in hypothyroid patients. It has been shown to return to normal after treatment with levothyroxine.

Leptin is another hormone that may also have a role in thyroid hormone, although this is controversial. Leptin is a hormone made in the body's fat cells and has a role in fat metabolism. Its function in weight control still needs to be determined. Working with your medical team to normalize thyroid hormone levels is the first step in weight control.

Insurance companies sometimes cover nutrition visits with a registered dietitian. Some insurance plans offer reduced rates for preferred providers, and some include only a copay. You should check to see what is offered by your insurance plan.

Staying Healthy with Hypothyroidism

If not in conflict with any other conditions, the recommendation for most people with hypothyroidism is a well-balanced diet. As there are potential problems with increased cholesterol and low-density lipoprotein levels (LDL), doctors and dietitians usually recommend a heart-healthy diet.

So what is a heart-healthy diet? The American Heart Association recommends limiting added sugar in the diet. Their recommendations are no more than 100 calories for women and no more than 150 calories for men from added sugar. Getting enough fiber is excellent (just remember to be careful about not having fiber at the same time your thyroid medication is taken). At least half of grains consumed should be in the form of whole grains.

FACT

Whole grains are not refined. They are made from all of the parts of the seed of the plant, called the kernel, or the "whole grain."

This includes the bran, germ, and endosperm of the grain. The following is a list of whole grains presented in order of consumption in the United States from the Agriculture Research Service Database:

- Whole wheat
- Whole oats/oatmeal
- Whole-grain corn
- Popcorn
- Brown rice
- Whole rye
- Whole-grain barley

- Wild rice
- Buckwheat
- Triticale
- Bulgur (cracked wheat)
- Millet
- Quinoa
- Sorghum

Lean protein is recommended as part of a heart-healthy diet. In addition to lean protein, oily fish should be consumed at least two times a week. Examples of heart-healthy fish include sardines, salmon, mackerel, and herring. Plant-based proteins should also be included in the diet. These foods include kidney beans, navy beans, black beans, and legumes. Grains such as quinoa are also sources of protein. Fatty meats should be limited, if consumed at all. Regular bacon, ground pork, pork spareribs, and processed sandwich meats such as bologna and hard salami are examples of fatty meats.

Saturated fats are not considered heart healthy. Recommendations by the American Heart Association include no more than 7 percent of calories from saturated fat. Trans fatty acids should be limited to no more than 1 percent of calories. In a 1,600-calorie diet, this is no more than a little over 2 grams.

FACT

According to the American Heart Association guidelines for a heart-healthy diet, 77 percent of all sodium consumed in the United States is from processed foods. Due to this statistic, it is recommended that over the next ten years food manufacturers and restaurants decrease the amount of added salt by 50 percent.

The American Heart Association recommendations for sodium have been lowered to 1,500 milligrams per day. As the recommendation has been lowered from 2,300 mg per day, they recommend Americans decrease consumption to 2,000 mg per day by the year 2013 and then decrease the amount to 1,500 mg per day by the year 2020.

As part of a heart-healthy diet, the American Heart Association recommends limiting the amount of beverages that contain added sugars and sweeteners that contain calories. Many beverages contain an excess of sugar. Most regular 12-ounce sodas contain 160–190 calories. These calories come from added sugar.

Exercise

When there is lack of energy and a lowered metabolism, it is not unusual for a person to stop exercising. Then, weight gain follows. Usually, it is recommended to get the thyroid hormone levels under control before you start an exercise program. The physician needs to be consulted to see if a stress test is necessary.

ESSENTIAL

A stress test may be done to make sure your heart is in good condition and that an exercise program will be tolerated. You may be asked not to consume food or beverages that contain caffeine for a day before. Usually, your heart and blood pressure are monitored while exercising on a treadmill or stationary bicycle.

You should ask if there are any restrictions on exercise. If there are restrictions, ask what can be done and if there is a cardiac rehabilitation center available. You can find programs that offer an individualized treatment plan to build up strength. The exercise is safely done in a monitored setting.

Working with a professional for exercise can help you establish what a good heart rate (beats/minute) should be as you exercise. They will teach you how to monitor your pulse rate as you exercise, and after. You should also learn proper exercise techniques for warm ups, workouts, and cool downs. If you have physician clearance to exercise, always ask what exercise is best. Usually, if there are no restrictions, a walking program is good to start. Using a pedometer or step counter is very helpful to monitor daily activity. Add steps every day as you can. Ten thousand steps a day is approximately 5 miles, and a goal that is recommended by many health care providers. If resistance exercise is recommended, do not use any equipment unless you have been properly trained to help prevent injury.

FACT

According to the American College of Sports Medicine, at least 60–90 minutes of exercise per day is necessary for many people to lose and maintain weight. They provide videos and specific exercise guidelines for Americans of all ages. Go to their website for help with an exercise program: *www.acsm.org/AM/Template.cfm?Section=Home_Page&TEMPLATE=CM/HTMLDisplay.cfm&CONTENTID=7764.*

Many patients complain that they just can't lose weight with hypothyroidism. The key to weight loss is proper thyroid levels, a healthy individualized diet plan, and the proper amount of exercise. When these key items are controlled, you will be ahead of the pack in maintaining your health!

CHAPTER 6

Diets for Autoimmune Thyroid Disease

A heart-healthy diet is usually recommended for autoimmune thyroid disease. The most common autoimmune thyroid diseases are Hashimoto's disease and Graves' disease. Unfortunately, it is not uncommon to have other autoimmune diseases coexisting with autoimmune thyroid disease. An autoimmune disease is when your body makes antibodies toward your own tissue. This can happen in many places in the body and cause many symptoms and coexisting dietary and medical needs. Depending on the other diseases, a heart-healthy diet may not be enough. You need to follow nutritional and dietary recommendations for all of your diseases. Do not be afraid to get help from your medical team, especially your registered dietitian. Knowing what to do about nutrition concerns of the comorbidities and following the recommended advice will play a large part in keeping yourself healthy.

The Possibility of Comorbidities

According to the American Autoimmune Related Disease Association, approximately one in five Americans have at least one of the 100 known autoimmune diseases. The two main thyroid diseases that are autoimmune are Graves' disease and Hashimoto's thyroiditis. Studies have indicated that approximately 25 percent of the people with Hashimoto's thyroiditis have other autoimmune diseases. Some of the diseases are more common in people with Hashimoto's disease and some are not seen as much.

Autoimmune thyroid disease and diseases such as type 1 diabetes and celiac disease are common. Other diseases such as Addison's disease, vitiligo, and systemic lupus erythematosus (SLE) have a correlation.

FACT

The American Autoimmune Related Disease Association has patient information on individual autoimmune diseases. Go to *www.aarda .org/patient_information.php* and look under "Patient Information." The pull-down menu has a list and explanation of many of the autoimmune diseases.

Pay attention to all of your comorbidities. They may have nutritional implications. Finding information that combines comorbidities is very rare but necessary. You need to take care of all of your conditions as a whole and feel comfortable eating what is healthy for you!

Type 1 Diabetes

Type 1 diabetes is an autoimmune disease where the body destroys the insulin-producing cells in the pancreas. Insulin is used by the body to move glucose (sugar) into cells, where it is processed and used for energy. When insulin is not present, the sugar cannot enter the cell from the blood stream and the blood sugar elevates, resulting in a high blood glucose level. The sugar also may "spill" into the urine. Weight loss occurs, despite eating to try to satisfy increased hunger. When sugar is high in the blood stream, you'll become very thirsty and will most likely drink more. The result is an increase in urination. Sometimes this is described as the three Ps of diabetes: polyphagia (increased hunger), polydipsia (increased thirst), and polyuria (increased urination). The body cannot be nourished because the sugar does not get into the cell to provide energy. When this happens, you will become very tired and irritable. Testing for type 1 diabetes includes measuring blood glucose levels and a test called a hemoglobin A1C that allows the medical team to evaluate the blood sugar control over the past 60–90 days. Type 1 diabetes is always treated with insulin.

FACT

People with type 2 diabetes do not have an autoimmune disease. Their bodies make insulin, but they may not be able to use the insulin they make, or they do not make enough insulin. Sometimes, controlling the amount of carbohydrates consumed that will turn into glucose is all that is needed. Others may need medication to help use the insulin they make or help them make more insulin. Others may need to take insulin. They may have thyroid disease at the same approximate rate as the general population.

The thyroid regulates the metabolism of carbohydrates and sugars in the body. In patients with hyperthyroidism, as the metabolism speeds up, they have more sugar absorbed by the intestine and also more released by the liver, due to the increased metabolism. Energy is wasted by the body due to inability to handle increased sugars. The term "thyroid diabetes" is used frequently to describe the effect that hyperthyroidism has on the control of diabetes. With increasing levels of thyroid hormone, insulin requirements also increase. When one has hypothyroidism, insulin requirements are decreased. If a patient has both thyroid disease and diabetes, the diabetes medication may need to be altered as the thyroid function is regulated.

Statistics show as many as 31 percent of women with type 1 diabetes have thyroid disease. Children and teenagers with type 1 diabetes have a higher incidence of hypothyroidism. There are also as many as 25 percent of women with type 1 diabetes that develop postpartum thyroiditis.

It is thought that in patients with type 2 diabetes with metabolic syndrome, there is a greater problem with subclinical hypothyroidism. According to the

American Heart Association, the metabolic syndrome is a condition with the following problems: increased abdominal fat, high cholesterol with an increase in the "bad" cholesterol (low density lipoproteins) and a decrease in the "good" cholesterol (high density lipoproteins). Triglycerides are often elevated in the blood work and there is an increase in blood pressure. Some of the medications used in controlling type 2 diabetes, such as some of the sulfonylureas and metformin, may affect thyroid hormone production in patients with hypothyroidism.

Thyroid screening has been recommended by the Endocrine Society and the American Thyroid Association in patients with diabetes. Due to the high incidence of thyroid disease in individuals with diabetes, the recipes in this book include the carbohydrate content and diabetes exchanges. If you have thyroid disease and diabetes, a registered dietitian (RD) and preferably a certified diabetes educator (CDE) should be consulted to help develop proper meal plans and provide nutrition counseling.

Celiac Disease

Celiac disease is an autoimmune disease characterized by intolerance to dietary gluten. The ingestion of gluten leads to an inflammatory response in the small intestine, which leads to damage to the villi. Villi are finger-like structures in the intestines that come in contact with nutrients for absorption into the body.

FACT

Symptoms of celiac disease include frequent bowel movements with fatty stools. Weight loss from malabsorption of food, fatigue, and anemia may also occur. Silent celiac disease is another manifestation in which symptoms are minimal. Early diagnosis can help prevent problems of malabsorption, such as anemia and osteoporosis.

The diagnosis of celiac disease is usually done by first screening for IgA antiendomysial antibodies and IgA antitissue transglutaminase antibodies (anti-tTG) in the blood. When positive, this may be followed by a small-intestine biopsy.

The incidence of celiac disease is greatly increased in people with auto-immune thyroid disease. Various studies show between 2–5 percent of people with these types of thyroid disorders also are afflicted with celiac disease. Reasoning for this is thought to be similar gene encoding. Patients with autoimmune thyroid disease might consider asking their doctor to screen for celiac disease if this has not been done.

ALERT

Individuals diagnosed with celiac disease with coexisting Hashimoto's disease should consider asking their physician about the proper dose of thyroid medication when starting the gluten-free diet. As the intestines heal, they may need their medication for hypothyroidism decreased due to better absorption. It is wise to monitor thyroid function at this time to avoid a swing from hypothyroidism to hyperthyroidism.

The gluten-free diet in patients with celiac disease may increase absorption of vitamins and minerals as well as calories. It is not unusual to gain weight as the villi heal. Sometimes weight gain is desirable and sometimes not. If it is not, it is advisable to ask your medical team to see a registered dietitian to develop an individualized meal plan. This meal plan needs to include ways to eat a healthy diet and eliminate gluten. Wheat, barley, and rye contain gluten. Unfortunately, there is a great deal of hidden gluten in many foods such as soy sauce, gravies, commercial broth, and processed foods, so this requires some care.

Most recipes in this book have suggestions on eliminating gluten if the recipe is not gluten free. Be sure to check all ingredients used to make sure they are gluten free. Many big food manufacturers will provide a list of gluten-free products they sell.

Be aware that even in some foods that do not list any gluten-containing components, food processing equipment may have previously been used for processing wheat, barley, or rye. This is commonly the case for many foods, such as nuts, which alone are gluten free but become cross contaminated when run through the mill. Oats are another concern. If planted in a field that a gluten-containing food has recently been grown in, a bit of that grain may be in the field with the oats. Therefore, it is necessary to buy gluten-free oats.

FACT

One company that will provide a list of their gluten-free products is Purdue Farms Incorporated. This way, you can know if the broth in their specific uncooked and cooked poultry products contains wheat or is gluten free. Call Purdue Farms Incorporated at 1-800-473-7383 to get a copy of this list.

IgA Nephropathy

IgA nephropathy, or Berger's disease, is an autoimmune kidney disease that causes nephritis or inflammation in the kidneys. Deposits of the antibody IgA collect in the kidney. One of the first symptoms seen is blood in the urine. This may progress to renal or kidney failure. Blood pressure medications and diuretics (water pills) may be part of the therapy.

ESSENTIAL

People with IgA nephropathy may be asked to reduce their sodium or salt intake. Fluid, protein, potassium, and phosphorus restrictions may also be needed if the disease progresses. End-stage renal failure may develop in one out of four patients with this condition. This usually happens over a period of up to twenty-five years.

Reviewing the literature, there are not as many references for coexisting IgA nephropathy and autoimmune thyroid disease as there are with type 1 diabetes or celiac disease, but it is a possibility. It is not uncommon to have more than one autoimmune disease. This is an autoimmune disease that has many nutritional restrictions. If you do have this or other kidney diseases, you may need the dietary information provided in this book.

There are many dietary changes that may develop with kidney disease. It is usually necessary to see a registered dietitian for understanding how to change your diet. Recipes in this book have values for sodium, protein, potassium, and phosphorus. These values many be needed to assess if the recipe can be enjoyed for IgA nephropathy as well as other kidney problems.

Ulcerative Colitis

It is thought that ulcerative colitis may be an autoimmune disease. It is one type of inflammatory bowel disease that affects the lower intestine and rectum, causing inflammation and at times severe cramping. It causes bloody diarrhea from ulcers that form, and the bleeding may cause anemia. There can also be loss of nutrients from the diarrhea as well as weight loss and fatigue. There have been documented cases of comorbidity of autoimmune thyroid disease with ulcerative colitis.

ESSENTIAL

The diet for ulcerative colitis may be very particular for each individual. It is important to work with a health care professional so that a nutritious meal plan can be developed. There may be foods that are usually thought of as healthy that cause distress when consumed.

It is thought that the immune system of individuals with ulcerative colitis react with bacteria that is in the digestive tract. Blood work and stool cultures help diagnose ulcerative colitis. A patient may also need a colonoscopy and sigmoidoscopy, so that samples of the colon can be examined.

Recording foods and how you feel after eating is very important. If certain foods cause pain and diarrhea, there may be healthy substitutes. Lactose, the natural sugar in milk, may be a problem. Talk to your dietitian about nutritious substitutions for milk, such as rice, almond, or soy milk.

In some people, high amounts of fiber may irritate the intestines in this condition. Asking the medical team how much fiber should be used is important. Sometimes it is raw fruits and vegetables that are irritating. Your food log will help you identify these problems so you can adjust your diet for the long term.

Foods that contain caffeine may also cause irritation, and coffee may affect the uptake of thyroid medication. Drinking adequate fluids is very important. Be sure to discuss proper amounts with your medical team.

Therapy and treatment of this condition may include prescription anti-inflammatory medications and steroids. If there is infection, it needs to be treated. Sometimes there are periods of long remission, but flair-ups may occur. Surgery may also be needed. Ask your medical team about all options.

Taking care of your complete health and dietary needs is very important. Talk to your medical team about using the meal plans in Appendix A as a part of your diet.

CHAPTER 7

Breakfast and Brunch

Apple-Cinnamon Smoothie

Applesauce is available in several versions; you can find chunky applesauce, smooth applesauce, and organic applesauce.

INGREDIENTS | SERVES 2

1 cup unsweetened applesauce

½ cup nonfat vanilla yogurt

½ teaspoon cinnamon

1 large apple, peeled and chopped

4 ice cubes

1. Place applesauce, yogurt, cinnamon, and apple in a blender or food processor and blend or process until smooth.

2. Add ice cubes and blend or process until thick. Pour into glasses and serve immediately.

PER SERVING: Calories: 156 | Protein: 3 g | Carbohydrates: 38 g | Fat: 0.4 g | Saturated Fat: 0.1 g | Cholesterol: 1 g | Sodium: 43 mg | Potassium: 320 mg | Phosphorus: 98 mg | Calcium: 119 mg | Fiber: 3 g | Exchanges: 2 Fruit, ½ Skim Milk | Gluten Free

Quinoa Berry Breakfast

Try other berries, nuts, or spices such as ginger or nutmeg to vary this nutritious breakfast cereal.

INGREDIENTS | SERVES 4

1 cup quinoa

2 cups water

¼ cup walnuts

1 teaspoon cinnamon

2 cups raw blackberries

Single-Serving Quick Tip

Use this basic recipe to make 4 servings at once. Refrigerate any leftover portions. Microwave 1–1½ minutes on high for single portions as needed. Use cooked quinoa within 3 days.

1. Rinse the quinoa in a fine-mesh sieve before cooking. Place quinoa, water, walnuts, and cinnamon in a 1½-quart saucepan and bring to a boil. Reduce heat to low, cover, and cook for 15 minutes, or until all water has been absorbed.

2. Add berries and serve with skim milk, soy milk, or sweetener, if desired.

PER SERVING: Calories Per Serving: 230 | Protein: 8 g | Carbohydrates: 36 g | Fat: 7.0 g | Saturated Fat: 0.7 g | Cholesterol: 0 mg | Sodium: 7 mg | Potassium: 388 mg | Phosphorus: 232 mg | Calcium: 57 mg | Fiber: 8 g | Exchanges: 1 Starch, 1½ Fruit, ½ Lean Meat, ½ Fat | Gluten Free

Cornmeal Grits

This warm cereal is similar to oatmeal. It can be eaten in a variety of ways: as a breakfast cereal, as a side with ham and eggs, or with cheese stirred in it and cooked and peeled shrimp on top.

INGREDIENTS | SERVES 4

4 cups water

½ teaspoon salt

1 cup polenta meal

2 tablespoons tub margarine (80 percent fat), unsalted

1. Put water and salt in a saucepan and bring to a boil.

2. Gradually add polenta and stir constantly over medium-low heat until it has thickened, about 15 minutes. Stir in margarine.

3. Serve immediately for soft grits or pour into a greased loaf pan and let cool. When cool, grits can be sliced and fried or grilled.

PER SERVING: Calories: 156 | Protein: 3 g | Carbohydrates: 24 g | Fat: 6.8 g | Saturated Fat: 1.2 g | Cholesterol: 0 g | Sodium: 311 mg | Potassium: 92 mg | Phosphorus: 74 mg | Calcium: 9 mg | Fiber: 2 g | Exchanges: 1½ Starch, 1 Fat | Gluten Free: Use gluten-free margarine

Baked Grapefruit

*Honey is the traditional sweetener for this treat. However,
the grapefruit is just as tasty with Splenda Brown caramelized on top.*

INGREDIENTS | SERVES 2

1 large grapefruit, halved and sectioned
2 tablespoons Splenda Brown
2 teaspoons (80% fat) tub margarine
4 small whole strawberries, for garnish

Grapefruit

Grapefruit is a wonderful, nutritious fruit. However, it does interfere with some medications. Ask your pharmacist if you have any problems with eating grapefruit.

1. Preheat oven to 400°F.

2. Place the grapefruit halves on a pan. Sprinkle with Splenda Brown, dot with buttery spread.

3. Bake for 10 minutes. Garnish with strawberries.

PER SERVING: Calories: 111 | Protein: 1 g | Carbohydrates: 15 g | Fat: 4.0 g | Saturated Fat: 0.7 g | Cholesterol: 0 g | Sodium: 1 mg | Potassium: 253 mg (approx.) | Phosphorus: 17 mg (approx.) | Calcium: 22 mg | Fiber: 2 g | Exchanges: 1 Fruit, 1 Fat | Gluten Free: Use gluten-free margarine

Simple and Skinny Cheese Omelet

For an even skinnier omelet, use fat-free cheese.

INGREDIENTS | SERVES 2

1 teaspoon olive oil

½ cup fat-free egg substitute

½ cup low-fat mozzarella shredded cheese

1. Heat the olive oil in a small skillet on low heat, then pour the egg substitute in to coat the surface. Cook until edges show firmness.

2. Sprinkle the cheese evenly over the egg mixture and fold one side over the other.

3. Flip the half-moon omelet so both sides are evenly cooked.

PER SERVING: Calories: 124 | Protein: 13 g | Carbohydrates: 2 g | Fat: 7.1 g | Saturated Fat: 3.4 g | Cholesterol: 15 g | Sodium: 229 mg | Potassium: 112 mg | Phosphorus: 148 mg | Calcium: 207 mg | Fiber: 0 g | Exchanges: 2 Lean Meat, ¼ Fat | Gluten Free: Substitute 4 egg whites for egg substitute. Use gluten-free mozzarella cheese.

Oatmeal

This is the comfort food of the high-fiber diet—warm, cozy, and delicious. This will keep a family going happily until lunch.

INGREDIENTS | SERVES 4

2 cups water
1 cup rolled oats
¼ teaspoon salt
½ cup dried currants
1 teaspoon ground cinnamon
1 cup sweetened almond milk, chilled

1. Bring water to a boil. Add the oats and salt and stir. Turn the heat to low and simmer 5 minutes.

2. Stir in the currants and simmer for 10 minutes, stirring occasionally.

3. Remove from heat and spoon cooked oatmeal into 4 bowls.

4. Sprinkle with ¼ teaspoon cinnamon.

5. Serve the cold almond milk on the side in a small pitcher.

PER SERVING: Calories: 151 | Protein: 4 g | Carbohydrates: 32 g | Fat: 2.0 g | Saturated Fat: 0.2 g | Cholesterol: 0 g | Sodium: 189 mg | Potassium: 283 mg | Phosphorus: 131 mg | Calcium: 86 mg | Fiber: 4 g | Exchanges: 2 Starch | Gluten Free: Use gluten-free oats

Buckwheat Pancakes

You can substitute almond milk for the cow's milk to deliver a slightly nutty flavor.

INGREDIENTS | SERVES 6

1 cup whole-wheat flour

½ cup buckwheat flour

1½ teaspoons low-sodium baking powder

2 egg whites from large eggs

¼ cup unsweetened apple juice concentrate

1¼ cup skim milk

What Is Buckwheat Flour?

You might think that buckwheat is part of the wheat family, but it's not. The flour actually comes from the seeds of a plant in the rhubarb family. It is gluten-free.

1. Sift the flours and baking powder together.

2. Combine the egg whites, apple juice concentrate, and skim milk.

3. Add the liquid mixture to the dry ingredients and mix well, but do not overmix. If necessary to reach the desired consistency, add ¼ cup extra skim milk.

4. Cook the pancakes in a nonstick skillet or on a griddle treated with nonstick spray over medium heat. Turn when pancakes start to form bubbles and cook until browned.

PER SERVING: Calories: 140 | Protein: 7 g | Carbohydrates: 29 g | Fat: 0.9 g | Saturated Fat: 0.2 g | Cholesterol: 1 mg | Sodium: 45 mg | Potassium 405 mg | Phosphorus 244 mg | Calcium: 130 mg | Fiber: 3 g | Exchanges: 2 Starch | Gluten Free: Replace whole-wheat flour with gluten-free all-purpose flour. Use gluten-free baking powder.

Vegetable Omelet

You could use other vegetables in this colorful omelet.
Chopped mushrooms, summer squash, or bell pepper would be delicious.

INGREDIENTS | SERVES 4

1 tablespoon olive oil
½ cup grated carrot
½ cup raw chopped broccoli
¼ cup finely chopped red onion
8 large egg whites
1 large egg yolk
¼ cup skim milk
1 teaspoon white pepper
½ cup grated Cheddar cheese

1. In a large nonstick skillet, heat olive oil over medium heat. Add carrot, broccoli, and onion and cook, stirring occasionally, until crisp-tender, about 4–5 minutes.

2. Meanwhile, in a medium bowl, beat egg whites until a soft foam forms. In a small bowl, combine the egg yolk with the milk and pepper and beat well. Fold the egg yolk mixture into the egg whites.

3. Pour the egg mixture into the pan. Cook, lifting the edges of the eggs so the uncooked mixture can flow underneath, until eggs are set but still moist.

4. Sprinkle with cheese, cover the pan, and cook for 1 minute. Uncover, fold omelet, and serve immediately.

PER SERVING: Calories: 152 | Protein: 13 g | Carbohydrates: 5 g | Fat: 9.4 g | Saturated Fat: 3.9 g | Cholesterol: 68 g | Sodium: 220 mg | Potassium: 245 mg | Phosphorus: 131 mg | Calcium: 144 mg | Fiber: 1 g | Exchanges: 1 Vegetable, 1½ Lean Meat, 1 Fat | Gluten Free

Peach and Raspberry Soufflé

Your guests should always be waiting for the soufflé, not vice versa.
This lower-fat soufflé is more delicate than the traditional version, so it may fall sooner.

INGREDIENTS | SERVES 4

1½ cups chopped frozen unsweetened peaches, thawed

2 tablespoons salted tub margarine

2 tablespoons white flour

½ teaspoon salt

¼ cup sugar, divided

3 tablespoons raspberry jelly

1 large egg yolk

6 large egg whites

¼ teaspoon cream of tartar

Garnishing

Soufflés and omelets can be garnished for added color and nutrition, too. Use ingredients that are in the recipe as garnishes. Whole raspberries would be a perfect garnish for the Peach and Raspberry Soufflé.

1. Preheat the oven to 400°F. Drain the peaches, reserving the juice.

2. In a medium pan, melt the margarine over medium heat. Add the flour and salt and cook and stir for 3 minutes, until bubbly.

3. Add 1 tablespoon sugar, the reserved peach juice, and jelly and stir until mixture bubbles and thickens.

4. Remove from heat and whisk in the egg yolk and drained peaches. Set aside.

5. In a large bowl, combine the remaining sugar with the egg whites and cream of tartar and beat until foamy. Gradually beat in remaining 3 tablespoons of sugar until stiff peaks form.

6. Stir a dollop of the egg-white mixture into the peach mixture, then fold in the remaining egg whites.

7. Spray the bottom of a 2-quart casserole dish with nonstick cooking spray and pour soufflé batter into the dish. Bake for 35–45 minutes, or until soufflé is puffed and deep golden brown. Serve immediately.

PER SERVING: Calories: 213 | Protein: 7 g | Carbohydrates: 35 g | Fat: 5.8 g | Saturated Fat: 1.3 g | Cholesterol: 53 g | Sodium: 436 mg | Potassium: 291 mg | Phosphorus: 49 mg | Calcium: 18 mg | Fiber: 1.7 g | Exchanges: 2 Fruit, 1 Lean Meat, ½ Fat | Gluten Free: Replace flour with gluten-free all-purpose flour. Use gluten-free cream of tartar and margarine.

Apple-Potato Pancakes

If you cant find pecans, substitute any of your favorite nuts!

INGREDIENTS | SERVES 4

½ cup potato granules

1½ cups boiling water

2 large whole eggs and 4 egg whites

2 teaspoons granulated sugar

½ teaspoon ground cinnamon

1 cup peeled and grated Granny Smith or Golden Delicious apple

¼ cup chopped pecans

Plain nonfat yogurt, sour cream, or applesauce (optional)

Fun Facts about Apples

Apples are a healthy choice in cooking. They are sodium, fat, and cholesterol free. They are a member of the rose family. George Washington had apple trees at Mount Vernon. Apples have five carpels (pockets) that contain seeds. There are more than 2,000 varieties of apples found in the United States alone.

1. To prepare the potatoes, add potato granules to a medium-sized bowl. Gradually pour the boiling water over the potato granules, whisking continuously to mix and whip.

2. In a small bowl, beat together the eggs, sugar, and cinnamon. Beat into the potatoes. Fold in the grated apple and chopped pecans.

3. Bring a nonstick skillet or griddle treated with nonstick spray to temperature over medium heat. (If using an electric griddle, preheat to 350°F–380°F.)

4. Cook the pancakes on both sides until golden brown. Serve hot, plain or topped with plain nonfat yogurt, sour cream, or applesauce.

PER SERVING: Calories: 217 | Protein: 10 g | Carbohydrates: 29 g | Fat: 7.6 g | Saturated Fat: 1.2 g | Cholesterol: 106 g | Sodium: 110 mg | Potassium: 327 mg | Phosphorus: 137 mg | Calcium: 39 mg | Fiber: 3 g | Exchanges: 1 Starch, 1 Fruit, 1 Lean Meat, ½ Fat | Gluten Free: Use gluten-free potato granules

Breakfast Pudding

Try substituting yellow squash for the zucchini—it's just as delicious, and still provides nutrition.

INGREDIENTS | SERVES 4

2 small zucchini, grated

1 small sweet onion, minced

1 clove garlic, minced

3 cups no-salt-added sweet corn (if fresh, cut from about 6 ears of corn)

6 small (5½" long) carrots, peeled and shredded

1 cup evaporated skim milk, divided

1 tablespoon unbleached all-purpose flour

1½ tablespoons cornmeal

1 cup (1% fat) cottage cheese

2 large eggs

½ teaspoon dried thyme

¼ teaspoon mustard powder

¼ teaspoon freshly ground black pepper

Canola spray oil with butter flavor

1 tablespoon bread crumbs

Start Your Day with Vegetables

According to the Centers for Disease Control and Prevention in the United States, only 14 percent of adults eat the recommended number of fruits and vegetables each day. Only 27 percent eat the recommended amount of three or more servings of vegetables per day.

1. Preheat oven to 325°F.

2. Add the zucchini, onion, garlic, corn, and carrots to a microwave-safe casserole dish. Cover and microwave on high for 3 minutes, then turn bowl and microwave on high for an additional 3 minutes. Leave the cover in place and set aside.

3. Whisk together ½ cup of milk, the flour, and cornmeal in a microwave-safe bowl and microwave on high for 1 minute. Whisk again and continue to microwave in 30-second increments, whisking between each time, until the mixture has thickened.

4. Combine the remaining ½ cup milk, the cottage cheese, eggs, thyme, mustard powder, and pepper in a blender or food processor and process until smooth and well mixed. Add the cottage cheese mixture to the corn mixture and stir to combine.

5. Treat an 11" × 7" oven-safe casserole dish with canola spray. Transfer the corn mixture to the casserole dish. Spread the cornmeal mixture over the top of the corn mixture. Sprinkle the bread crumbs over the top. Spray lightly with the canola oil.

6. Bake for 1 hour. Let stand for 5 minutes. Serve hot.

PER SERVING: Calories: 300 | Protein: 21 g | Carbohydrates: 46 g | Fat: 5.5 g | Saturated Fat: 1.6 g | Cholesterol: 111 g | Sodium: 382 mg | Potassium: 897 mg | Phosphorus: 419 mg | Calcium: 276 mg | Fiber: 5 g | Exchanges: 2 Starch, ½ Skim Milk, 2 Vegetable, 1 Lean Meat | Gluten Free: Use gluten-free bread crumbs, flour, and cooking spray

Eggs Benedict

This can be made vegetarian by substituting grilled portobello mushrooms for the Canadian bacon.

INGREDIENTS | SERVES 4

1 ounce evaporated skim milk

½ cup low-fat mayonnaise

2 teaspoons lemon juice

4 medium eggs

4 slices Canadian bacon

2 whole-wheat regular-sized English muffins

Cayenne pepper or paprika to garnish (optional)

Eggs Benedict with Vegetables

Many vegetables can be added to this dish. To make this even more delicious, steam some green beans, asparagus, or spinach and add as the first ingredient on your English muffin.

1. Mix the skim milk with the mayonnaise and lemon juice and heat in the microwave for about 40 seconds to warm.

2. Crack each egg into individual microwaveable bowls, being careful not to break the yolks.

3. Cover each bowl with plastic wrap and microwave on high until the whites are cooked and yolks firm, about 2 minutes.

4. In a skillet, cook the bacon. Toast the muffins in the toaster.

5. Place the bacon on the whole-wheat muffin pieces.

6. Add the eggs on the bacon and top each egg with 2 tablespoons of mayonnaise mixture. Sprinkle with paprika.

PER SERVING: Calories: 248 | Protein: 14 g | Carbohydrates: 20 g | Fat: 12.9 g | Saturated Fat: 3.1 g | Cholesterol: 207 g | Sodium: 691 mg | Potassium: 234 mg | Phosphorus: 198 mg | Calcium: 100 mg | Fiber: 1 g | Exchanges: 1 Starch, 2 Lean Meat, 1½ Fat | Gluten Free: Use gluten-free English muffins and mayonnaise

Toad in a Hole

In Britain, Toad in a Hole involves baking sausages and Yorkshire pudding in a large pan with bacon-fat drippings and flour, but this recipe—a Pennsylvania Dutch favorite—is far simpler and far less fattening.

INGREDIENTS | SERVES 1

1 slice of approximately 80-calorie bread, any kind

1 large egg

Salt and pepper, to taste

Flipping Toads

As it cooks, the egg adheres to the bread. This makes it super simple to flip the bread in the pan without worrying about dislodging the egg. Be sure to flip your eggs after they've had time to set. Otherwise, you risk getting runny egg all over the place, which won't affect taste but will leave you with a mess.

1. Use a circular cookie cutter to cut a hole in the center of a slice of bread.

2. Place on a warm skillet, sprayed lightly with nonfat cooking spray.

3. Crack the egg and put it in the hole in the bread.

4. Fry and flip to desired consistency.

5. Add salt and pepper, to taste.

PER SERVING Calories: 151 | Protein: 9 g | Carbohydrates: 16 g | Fat: 6.0 g | Saturated Fat: 01.7 g | Cholesterol: 211 g | Sodium: 252 mg | Potassium: 212 mg | Phosphorus: 169 mg | Calcium: 53 mg | Fiber: 2 g | Exchanges: 1 Starch, 1 Lean Meat, ½ Fat | Gluten Free: Use gluten-free bread

Soft Polenta and Peas

This is a savory breakfast with a touch of sweetness from the peas.
You can add sweet winter squash, carrots, corn, or lemon juice for variety.

INGREDIENTS | SERVES 4

1 cup regular enriched corn grits
4 cups water
¼ teaspoon salt
½ cup frozen peas

What Is Polenta?

Polenta is corn meal mush or corn grits. It is used in many recipes to add versatility.

1. In a saucepan, toast corn grits until fragrant. Add water and salt.

2. Bring to a boil, lower the heat, and simmer, covered, for 20 minutes. Stir polenta occasionally.

3. Add peas and continue to cook until hot.

PER SERVING Calories per serving: 209 | Protein: 5 g | Carbohydrates: 38 g | Fat: 4.1 g | Saturated Fat: 0.6 g | Cholesterol: 0 g | Sodium: 172 mg | Potassium: 112 mg | Phosphorus: 91 mg | Calcium: 83 mg | Fiber: 3 g | Exchanges: 2½ Starch | Gluten Free

CHAPTER 8

Appetizers

Pear, Roquefort, and Walnuts on Endive

This appetizer gets fiber from the endive lettuce petals, pears, and walnuts, which are partnered with blue cheese in a classic combination of flavors.

INGREDIENTS | SERVES 6

2 heads Belgian endive
2 large ripe Asian pears
2 ounces Roquefort cheese
¼ cup chopped walnuts

1. Separate the leaves of the endive and trim the stem ends. Lay the leaves out on a tray.

2. Core and slice the pears and lay a slice on each endive leaf.

3. Crumble a little Roquefort cheese onto the pear slices and sprinkle them with walnuts. Serve immediately.

PER SERVING: Calories: 109 | Protein: 3 g | Carbohydrates: 11 g | Fat: 6.4 g | Saturated Fat: 2.1 g | Cholesterol: 9 mg | Sodium: 171 mg | Potassium: 179 mg | Phosphorus: 69 mg | Calcium: 75 mg | Fiber: 4 g | Exchanges: 1 Fruit, ½ Lean Meat, ½ Fat | Gluten Free: Use gluten-free cheese

Roasted Garlic and Red Pepper Hummus

Use sweet potato chips to dip for an extra treat!

INGREDIENTS | SERVES 8

2 cloves roasted garlic

2 cups cooked (without salt or fat) garbanzo beans, drained

⅓ cup tahini

⅓ cup lemon juice

½ cup chopped roasted red peppers

¼ teaspoon dried basil

¼ teaspoon freshly ground black pepper, to taste

1. In a food processor, combine the roasted garlic, garbanzo beans, tahini, lemon juice, roasted red peppers, and basil. Process until the mixture is smooth.

2. Season to taste with freshly ground pepper and transfer to a covered bowl and chill until ready to serve.

PER SERVING: Calories: 139 | Protein: 6 g | Carbohydrates: 16 g | Fat: 6.6 g | Saturated Fat: 0.9 g | Cholesterol: 0 mg | Sodium: 7 mg | Potassium: 200 mg | Phosphorus: 146 mg | Calcium: 39 mg | Fiber: 4 g | Exchanges: 1 Starch, ½ Lean Meat, ½ Fat | Gluten Free: Use gluten-free tahini

Fruit Cup with Creamy Dressing

Garnish with a few nuts to add additional crunch and protein.

INGREDIENTS | SERVES 2

⅛ cup peeled and grated carrots

10 seedless raisins

¼ of a small apple, sliced

6 seedless red or green grapes

4 ounces plain nonfat yogurt

1 tablespoon unsweetened, no-salt-added applesauce

1 teaspoon lemon juice

¼ teaspoon honey

⅛ teaspoon pumpkin pie spice

⅛ teaspoon finely grated fresh lemon zest

1. Arrange the carrots and fruit in a small cup.

2. Mix the yogurt, applesauce, lemon juice, honey, and pumpkin pie spice together and drizzle over the fruit. Sprinkle lemon zest over the top.

PER SERVING: Calories: 66 | Protein: 4 g | Carbohydrates: 14 g | Fat: 0.2 g | Saturated Fat: 0.1 g | Cholesterol: 1 mg | Sodium: 51 mg | Potassium: 237 mg | Phosphorus: 98 mg | Calcium: 124 mg | Fiber: 1 g | Exchanges: ½ Fruit, ½ Skim Milk | Gluten Free

Mushroom Caviar

Refrigerated leftovers will last a few days. Spread on toasted bread and pop under the broiler for 1 or 2 minutes for tasty mushroom-garlic toast.

INGREDIENTS | SERVES 12

1½ cups portobello mushrooms

1½ cups white button mushrooms

¼ cup chopped scallions

4 cloves dry-roasted garlic

1 teaspoon fresh lemon juice

½ teaspoon balsamic vinegar

1 tablespoon extra-virgin olive oil

½ teaspoon fresh, chopped thyme (optional)

Sea salt and freshly ground black pepper, to taste (optional)

Pseudo-Sauté

When onions and scallions are sautéed in butter or oil, they go through a caramelization process that doesn't occur when they're steamed. To create this flavor without increasing the fat in a recipe, transfer steamed vegetables to a nonstick wok or skillet (coated with nonstick spray or a small portion of the oil called for in the recipe) and sauté until the extra moisture evaporates.

1. Cut the portobello mushrooms into ¼" cubes. Cut the white button mushrooms into halves or quarters. (The mushroom pieces should be roughly uniform in size.)

2. Place the mushrooms and chopped scallion in a microwave-safe bowl, cover, and microwave on high for 1 minute. Rotate the bowl and continue to microwave in 30-second intervals until tender.

3. Transfer the scallions and mushrooms to a food processor. (Reserve any liquid to use for thinning the "caviar," if necessary.) Pulse the food processor several times to chop the mixture, scraping down the sides of the bowl as needed.

4. Add the remaining ingredients and pulse until mixed. Place in a small crock or serving bowl, and serve warm.

PER SERVING: Calories: 17 | Protein: 1 g | Carbohydrates: 1 g | Fat: 1.2 g | Saturated Fat: 0.2 g | Cholesterol: 0 mg | Sodium: 2 mg | Potassium: 77.5 mg | Phosphorus: 22 mg | Calcium: 4 mg | Fiber: 0.3 g | Exchanges: 1 Free Exchange | Gluten Free

Super Spicy Salsa

Salsa can be used in so many ways.
It's delicious as a garnish for chili or grilled chicken.

INGREDIENTS | SERVES 14

2 jalapeño peppers, minced

1 habanero pepper, minced

1 large green bell pepper, minced

4 cloves garlic, minced

1 medium red onion, chopped

5 large ripe tomatoes, chopped (1 large tomato weighs 7 ounces)

3 tablespoons lemon juice

¼ teaspoon salt

½ teaspoon white pepper

¼ cup chopped fresh cilantro

1. In a large bowl, combine jalapeños, habanero pepper, bell pepper, garlic, red onion, and tomatoes.

2. In a small bowl, combine lemon juice, salt, and pepper and stir to dissolve salt. Add to tomato mixture along with cilantro.

3. Cover and refrigerate for 3–4 hours before serving.

PER SERVING: Calories: 28 | Protein: 1 g | Carbohydrates: 6 g | Fat: 0.2 g | Saturated Fat: 0.0 g | Cholesterol: 0 mg | Sodium: 50 mg | Potassium: 250 mg | Phosphorus: 31 mg | Calcium: 17 mg | Fiber: 1 g | Exchanges: 1 Vegetable | Gluten Free

Pepper Heat

The heat in a pepper is concentrated in its seeds and inner membranes. If you prefer a milder taste, just remove and discard the seeds and membranes before mincing. Remember, the smaller the pepper the hotter. Habaneros and Scotch bonnet peppers are some of the hottest, while pepperoncini and poblano peppers are milder.

Grilled Cherry Tomatoes with Parmesan Cheese

When cherry tomatoes are grilled, their flavor is intensified.
Each little tomato will burst with flavor in your mouth.

INGREDIENTS | SERVES 6

24 cherry tomatoes
1 tablespoon extra-virgin olive oil
1 tablespoon red wine vinegar
¼ teaspoon salt
Pinch white pepper
1 tablespoon chopped fresh mint
2 tablespoons shaved Parmesan cheese

1. Tear off an 18" × 12" sheet of heavy-duty aluminum foil. Poke cherry tomatoes with the tip of a knife (to prevent splitting) and arrange on foil.

2. In a small bowl, combine oil, vinegar, salt, and pepper and mix well. Spoon over tomatoes.

3. Bring together foil edges and fold over several times, sealing the package. Leave some room for expansion during cooking.

4. Prepare and preheat grill. Grill the foil packet over medium coals for 4–6 minutes, or until tomatoes are hot.

5. Remove from grill, open package, and sprinkle with mint and shaved Parmesan. Serve immediately.

PER SERVING: Calories: 42 | Protein: 1 g | Carbohydrates: 3 g | Fat: 2.9 g | Saturated Fat: 0.6 g | Cholesterol: 1 mg | Sodium: 132 mg | Potassium: 158 mg | Phosphorus: 29 mg | Calcium: 27 mg | Fiber: 1 g | Exchanges: ½ Vegetable, ½ Fat | Gluten Free

Stuffed Eggs with Salmon Mousse

Put the salmon mixture into a cake-decorating bag and pipe it into the egg whites for a beautiful presentation.

INGREDIENTS | SERVES 12

4 ounces boneless cold-smoked salmon

1 (3-ounce) package light cream cheese, softened

¼ cup low-fat mayonnaise

¼ teaspoon pepper

2 tablespoons chopped chives

12 hard-cooked eggs, halved, yolks removed

2 cups curly parsley

Hard-Cooked Eggs

To hard-cook eggs, place large eggs in a saucepan and cover with cold water. Bring to a boil over high heat. When water is boiling furiously, cover pan, remove from heat, and let stand for 15 minutes. Then place the saucepan in the sink and run cold water into it until the eggs feel cold. Crack shells under water, then peel the eggs.

1. In a blender or food processor, combine salmon, cream cheese, mayonnaise, and pepper. Blend or process until smooth. Stir in chives.

2. Fill egg white halves with the salmon mixture. Arrange on parsley on a serving plate. Cover with plastic wrap and chill for 2 hours before serving.

PER SERVING: Calories: 60 | Protein: 6 g | Carbohydrates: 2 g | Fat: 2.7 g | Saturated Fat: 1.1 g | Cholesterol: 7 mg | Sodium: 231 mg | Potassium: 133 mg | Phosphorus: 36 mg | Calcium: 26 mg | Fiber: 0 g | Exchanges: 1 Lean Meat | Gluten Free: use gluten-free cream cheese and mayonnaise

Fried Green Tomatoes with Goat Cheese

*Make sure the tomatoes are really green, with no touch of red, for best results.
Serve these hot with a knife and fork.*

INGREDIENTS | SERVES 8

3 large green tomatoes
1 large egg
¼ cup nonfat buttermilk
½ cup yellow cornmeal
¼ cup all-purpose flour
1 teaspoon low-sodium baking powder
⅛ teaspoon cayenne pepper
½ cup virgin olive oil
2 ounces soft goat cheese

Frying Foods

When frying at the correct temperature, food absorbs approximately 8–25 percent of the oil. If the pan is not hot it will absorb more. If it is too hot, it will smoke and burn. For this recipe calculation, 25 percent of the oil was used.

1. Cut tomatoes into ⅓" slices and discard ends.

2. In a shallow bowl, combine egg and buttermilk and whisk to combine.

3. On a plate, combine cornmeal, flour, baking powder, and pepper and mix well.

4. Place olive oil in a large saucepan over medium heat. When hot, dip tomato slices into egg mixture, then into cornmeal mixture to coat. Place carefully in oil and fry, turning once, until golden brown, about 3–5 minutes per side.

5. Drain fried tomatoes on paper towels and top each with a bit of goat cheese. Serve immediately.

PER SERVING: Calories: 134 | Protein: 5 g | Carbohydrates: 15 g | Fat: 6.4 g | Saturated Fat: 1.9 g | Cholesterol: 30 mg | Sodium: 5 mg | Phosphorus: 128 mg | Calcium: 59 mg | Fiber: 2 g | Exchanges: 1 Starch, 1 Fat | Gluten Free: Use gluten-free all-purpose flour, baking powder, and cornmeal

Picnic Breakfast Stuffed Hard-Boiled Eggs

These stuffed eggs travel beautifully and make any picnic special. Enjoy them as an appetizer anywhere— at the beach, on a mountain top, or in the car. Do make sure you put them in your cooler.

INGREDIENTS | SERVES 6

½ cup flaked crabmeat (not packed)

¼ cup light mayonnaise

Juice of ½ lemon

½ teaspoon Old Bay seasonings or chili powder

6 large hardboiled eggs, halved, yolks removed from whites

1 teaspoon Worcestershire sauce

½ teaspoon dried dill weed

Dash of ground black pepper

1. Mix the crabmeat, mayonnaise, lemon juice, and Old Bay seasoning or chili powder.

2. Set cooked egg white halves on a serving platter.

3. Mash the egg yolks with a fork. Mix the yolks with the crabmeat mixture and Worcestershire sauce. Pile on the egg whites. Sprinkle with dill weed and pepper.

4. Wrap stuffed eggs individually with foil if packing for a picnic. Or serve on a platter, with cucumber slices separating stuffed eggs to keep them from rolling around.

PER SERVING: Calories: 123 | Protein: 9 g | Carbohydrates: 2 g | Fat: 8.8 g | Saturated Fat: 2.2 g | Cholesterol: 225 mg | Sodium: 169 mg | Potassium: 133 mg | Phosphorus: 114 mg | Calcium: 47 mg | Fiber: 0 g | Exchanges: 1½ Lean Meat, ½ Fat | Gluten Free: Use gluten-free Worcestershire sauce and mayonnaise

Miniature Crab Cakes

Traditionally, crab cakes are fried in butter. This healthy alternative bakes them. It also takes advantage of panko, a type of bread crumb that adds a lot of crunch to a dish without adding a lot of fat.

INGREDIENTS | SERVES 6

8 ounces crabmeat

¼ cup light mayonnaise

Juice and zest of ½ lemon

1 large egg

1 tablespoon Chili Sauce

2 tablespoons sweet white onion, minced

1 teaspoon dried dill weed or 1 tablespoon fresh dill, snipped

1 teaspoon dry Dijon-style mustard blended with 2 teaspoons water

½ cup panko

1. Preheat the oven to 450°F. Prepare a baking sheet with nonstick spray.

2. Mix the first 8 ingredients together in a bowl.

3. Spread the panko bread crumbs on a piece of waxed paper.

4. Make 12 little burgers using about 1 tablespoonful of the crab mixture. Coat with panko.

5. Bake for 5 minutes. Turn and bake for another 5 minutes, or until very crisp. Serve on slices of cucumber, leaves of romaine lettuce, or small pieces of bread.

PER SERVING: Calories: 102 | Protein: 7 g | Carbohydrates: 10 g | Fat: 4 g | Saturated Fat: 1g | Cholesterol: 20 mg | Sodium: 270 mg | Potassium: 170 mg | Phosphorus: 77 mg | Calcium: 42 mg | Fiber: 1 g | Exchanges: ½ Starch, 1 Lean Meat | Gluten Free: Replace panko with gluten-free crumbs, use gluten-free mayonnaise, chili sauce, and mustard

Snacks Versus Treats

A snack is a small part of a healthy diet, something you can eat every day to maintain well-being. Snacks include fruit, raw veggies, cheese and crackers, and if calories allow, even a half-sandwich. A treat is something you have rarely on special occasions. Treats include cookies, cakes, candy, and ice cream.

Mini Pizzas with Broccoli and Cheese

If you are out of tomato sauce, substitute ¾ cup low-sodium tomato paste mixed with 1 cup water.

INGREDIENTS | SERVES 8

4 whole-wheat English muffins
1 cup low-sodium tomato sauce
1 teaspoon dried oregano
1 teaspoon cayenne pepper, or to taste
½ pound broccoli florets, chopped and blanched
8 (1-ounce) slices low-fat mozzarella cheese
¼ cup finely grated low-sodium Parmesan cheese

Endless Pizza Variations

You can make pizza with spinach, asparagus, peppers, or whatever you like. Most kids will eat their veggies when incorporated into a pizza.

1. Preheat your oven to 450°F.

2. Prepare a cookie sheet with nonstick spray.

3. Place English muffin halves on sheet and spread 2 tablespoons of tomato sauce on each. Sprinkle with oregano and cayenne. Spread with broccoli, then add the mozzarella.

4. Sprinkle with Parmesan and bake for 15 minutes, or until the crust is nicely browned.

PER SERVING: Calories: 189 | Protein: 14 g | Carbohydrates: 21 g | Fat: 6.8 g | Saturated Fat: 3.8 g | Cholesterol: 18 mg | Sodium: 259 mg | Potassium: 429 mg | Phosphorus: 297 mg | Calcium: 313 mg | Fiber: 5 g | Exchanges: 1 Starch, 1 Vegetable, 1 Lean Meat, ½ Fat | Gluten Free: Use gluten-free English muffins

CHAPTER 9

Soups and Stews

Chilled Cucumber Soup

Apple cider vinegar may be substituted for the red wine vinegar

INGREDIENTS | SERVES 4

2 large cucumbers, peeled, seeded, and chopped

1 ounce apple juice concentrate

1 tablespoon red wine vinegar

1½ cups cold, cultured 1% low-fat buttermilk

Dried dill weed and lemon zest (optional)

1. Place the cucumbers, apple juice concentrate, and vinegar in a food processor. Process briefly, then add the buttermilk and process again until smooth.

2. Cover and refrigerate until ready to serve. Serve chilled with a pinch of dried dill weed and some lemon zest floating on top of each serving, if desired.

PER SERVING: Calories: 67 | Protein: 4 g | Carbohydrates: 11 g | Fat: 1.0 g | Saturated Fat: 0.5 g | Cholesterol: 3.7 mg | Sodium: 100 mg | Potassium: 364 mg | Phosphorus: 114 mg | Calcium: 129 mg | Fiber: 1 g | Exchanges: ½ Skim Milk, 1 Vegetable | Gluten Free

Chicken Corn Chowder

Boneless turkey breast can be substituted for the skinless chicken.

INGREDIENTS | SERVES 10

1 pound boneless, skinless chicken breast, cut into chunks

1 large onion, chopped

1 medium red bell pepper, diced

1 large potato, diced (flesh only)

2 (16-ounce) cans reduced-sodium chicken broth

1 (8¾-ounce) can unsalted cream-style corn

½ cup all-purpose flour

2 cups skim milk

4 ounces low-fat Cheddar cheese, diced

½ teaspoon sea salt

½ teaspoon freshly ground pepper

½ cup processed vegetarian bacon bits

Why Is Homemade Soup Usually Healthier Than Canned Soup?

You have control of the ingredients. Some canned soups have more than 1000 mg of sodium in 1 cup. Reduce this by comparing ingredients and selecting the healthiest before adding them.

1. Spray a large soup pot with nonstick cooking spray and heat on medium setting until hot. Add the chicken, onion, and bell pepper and sauté over medium heat, stirring until the chicken is browned on all sides and the vegetables are tender, about 15.

2. Stir in the potatoes and broth and bring to a boil. Reduce the heat and simmer, covered, for 20 minutes.

3. Stir in the corn.

4. Blend the flour and milk in a bowl, then gradually stir it into the pot. Increase heat to medium and cook until the mixture comes to a boil, then reduce heat and simmer until soup is thickened, stirring constantly.

5. Add the cheese and stir until it's melted and blended into the soup. Add the salt and pepper, and sprinkle with bacon bits before serving.

PER SERVING: Calories: 195 | Protein: 17 g | Carbohydrates: 23 g | Fat: 4.0 g | Saturated Fat: 1.1 g | Cholesterol: 25 mg | Sodium: 376 mg | Potassium: 540 mg | Phosphorus: 263 mg | Calcium: 129 mg | Fiber: 2 g | Exchanges: 1 Starch, 1 Vegetable, 1½ Lean Meat | Gluten Free: Use gluten-free flour and broth

White Bean, Sausage, and Escarole Soup

This is filling and tasty, a good home-style country soup.
Serve it with a whole-grain bread toasted and drizzled with olive oil and a crisp salad on the side.

INGREDIENTS | SERVES 6

6 ounces Italian sweet turkey sausage

2¼ cups water

2 tablespoons olive oil

4 cloves garlic, minced

2 medium onions, chopped

2 (14-ounce) cans no-salt diced tomatoes, undrained

1 cup cooked Great Northern white beans without salt or fat added

1 cup cooked lima beans without salt or fat added

3 cups low-sodium beef broth

2 cups water

6 cups chopped escarole

1 teaspoon dried oregano

1 cup parsley, chopped

⅓ cup grated Parmesan cheese

Cooking and Freezing Dry Beans ahead of Time Saves Time!

Soak, sort, and cook beans according to package directions and without salt. If you can gently squeeze beans between your fingers, they are done. Drain beans and then cool in the refrigerator. Label and date a freezer bag or container and freeze in batches that are the right size for your recipes. Thaw in the refrigerator when ready to use.

1. Place sausage in a soup pot over medium heat. Add ¼ cup water and bring to a simmer. Simmer sausage, turning occasionally, until water evaporates. Then cook, turning frequently, until browned. Remove from pot and discard drippings; do not wash pot. Cut sausage into ½" slices.

2. Add olive oil to pot and add garlic and onion. Cook and stir until tender, about 5 minutes.

3. Add tomatoes and stir. Add beans to pot along with broth, 2 cups water, escarole, and oregano. Simmer for 15–25 minutes, until escarole is tender.

4. Add sausage and parsley and simmer for 5 minutes. Serve each soup bowl with a sprinkling of Parmesan cheese.

PER SERVING: Calories: 240 | Protein: 15 g | Carbohydrates: 27 g | Fat: 9.4 g | Saturated Fat: 2.7 g | Cholesterol: 16 mg | Sodium: 357 mg | Potassium: 938 mg | Phosphorus: 257 mg | Calcium: 184 mg | Fiber: 8 g | Exchanges: 1 Starch, 2½ Vegetable, 1 Lean Meat, 1 Fat | Gluten Free: Use gluten-free sausage and broth

Chunky Irish Potato-Leek Soup

Versions of this soup have nourished generations. The onion and leek become sweet through long cooking, and the potatoes add a rich heartiness.

INGREDIENTS | SERVES 6

2 tablespoons olive oil

2 leeks, sliced

2 medium onions, chopped

2 tablespoons flour

3 cups low-sodium chicken broth

1 cup water

6 medium Yukon Gold potatoes, chopped

⅛ teaspoon cayenne pepper

1 cup 1% milk

1 cup fat-free half-and-half

¼ teaspoon nutmeg

½ cup chives, minced

¼ cup chopped parsley

Preparing Leeks

Leeks are a large, mild member of the onion family. They can be difficult to prepare because they are grown in sandy soil, and sand gets in between all the layers. To prepare, slice leeks in half lengthwise, then cut into ¼" slices. Place in a large bowl of cold water and swish with your hands so the sand falls to the bottom of the bowl.

1. In a large soup pot, heat olive oil over medium heat and add sliced leeks and onion. Cook and stir for 5 minutes.

2. Blend in flour and cook and stir for 3 minutes, until bubbly.

3. Add broth, water, and potatoes. Bring to a simmer, then reduce heat to low, cover, and simmer for 15–20 minutes, or until potatoes are tender. Mash some of the potatoes with a potato masher, leaving some whole.

4. Stir in cayenne pepper, milk, half-and-half, and nutmeg and heat until soup steams. Add chives and parsley, and serve immediately.

PER SERVING: Calories: 291 | Protein: 10 g | Carbohydrates: 51 g | Fat: 6.6 g | Saturated Fat: 1.6 g | Cholesterol: 4 mg | Sodium: 135 mg | Potassium: 1251 mg | Phosphorus: 295 mg | Calcium: 148 mg | Fiber: 7 g | Exchanges: 3 Starch, 1 Vegetable, ½ Fat | Gluten Free: Use gluten-free flour and broth

Ratatouille

This rich vegetable stew can be served over brown rice, pasta, or couscous, either hot or cold.

INGREDIENTS | SERVES 6

2 tablespoons olive oil

2 medium onions, chopped

4 cloves garlic, minced

1 medium green bell pepper, sliced

1 large yellow bell pepper, sliced

1¼ pounds eggplant, peeled and cubed

¼ teaspoon salt

¼ teaspoon pepper

2 tablespoons flour

2 medium zucchini, sliced

1 tablespoon red wine vinegar

2 tablespoons capers, rinsed

¼ cup chopped flat-leaf parsley

1. In a large saucepan, heat olive oil over medium heat. Add onion and garlic and cook and stir until crisp-tender, about 3 minutes.

2. Add bell peppers and cook and stir until crisp-tender, about 3 minutes.

3. Sprinkle eggplant with salt, pepper, and flour. Add to saucepan and cook and stir until eggplant begins to soften, about 10–15 minutes.

4. Add remaining ingredients except parsley, cover, and simmer for 30–35 minutes, or until vegetables are soft and mixture is blended. Sprinkle with parsley and serve.

PER SERVING: Calories: 110 | Protein: 3 g | Carbohydrates: 16 g | Fat: 5.0 g | Saturated Fat: 0.7 g | Cholesterol: 0 mg | Sodium: 195 mg | Potassium: 528 mg | Phosphorus: 74 mg | Calcium: 40 mg | Fiber: 5 g | Exchanges: 3 Vegetable, 1 Fat | Gluten Free: Use gluten-free flour

Eggplant

Eggplant is very low in calories and sodium and has a fairly high fiber content, about 2 grams per cup. It has lots of minerals, but a low vitamin content. It does contain the phytochemical monoterpene, which may help prevent cancer. To reduce bitterness, choose smaller eggplants that are firm and heavy for their size.

Black Bean Soup

You can use canned black beans to make this recipe immediately or soak dried beans and then cook them before starting this recipe. Traditional garnishes for black bean soup include shredded Cheddar cheese and sour cream.

INGREDIENTS | SERVES 6

¼ cup minced shallots

2 tablespoons olive oil

1 large potato, peeled and diced

4 cups low-sodium chicken broth

2 cups cooked black beans (made without adding salt)

1 teaspoon dried thyme

½ teaspoon ground coriander

½ ounce dry sherry

1 teaspoon salt

6 lemon slices (from 1 large lemon)

2 tablespoons chopped chives

1. Sauté shallots in olive oil. Add potato and chicken broth and simmer for 30 minutes.

2. Add black beans, thyme, and coriander and simmer 45 minutes.

3. Purée ⅛ of the soup in a blender and return it to the pot.

4. Stir in the sherry and salt.

5. Serve hot, garnished with lemon slices and chives.

PER SERVING: Calories: 200 | Protein: 10 g | Carbohydrates: 29 g | Fat: 5.9 g | Saturated Fat: 1.0 g | Cholesterol: 0 mg | Sodium: 441 mg | Potassium: 652 mg | Phosphorus: 171 mg | Calcium: 42 mg | Fiber: 7 g | Exchanges: 2 Starch, ½ Lean Meat, ½ Fat | Gluten Free: Use gluten-free broth

Soaking Beans

To help keep the gas factor down, dried beans need a soak. Fill a saucepan with 1½ quarts water and add 1 cup beans. Bring the water and beans to a boil and simmer for 2 minutes. Turn the heat off and let the beans sit in the water overnight, at least 8 hours. Most of the gas-causing elements will dissolve into the water. Discard the soaking water and add fresh water to cook the beans.

Harvest Stew

*Add fresh herbs from the garden to this soup to suit your taste,
and throw in any extra vegetables you may have on hand.*

INGREDIENTS | SERVES 6

1 pound stewing beef cubes, lean and trimmed of fat

2 tablespoons olive oil

¼ cup flour

¾ cup diced onions

½ cup sliced carrots

½ cup diced celery

1 leek, cleaned and diced

6 garlic cloves, peeled

2 cups diced zucchini

1 large potato, peeled and diced

3 turnips, diced

2 large tomatoes, chopped

1 bay leaf

3 sprigs fresh thyme

4 cups low-sodium beef broth

2 tablespoons Worcestershire sauce

Pepper, to taste

1. Brown the beef cubes in olive oil. Sprinkle the flour over the meat and stir to coat and distribute.

2. Add the onions, carrots, celery, leek, garlic, zucchini, potato, turnips, tomatoes, bay leaf, thyme sprigs, and beef broth. Bring to a boil, then lower the heat and simmer for 60 minutes.

3. Remove the bay leaf and thyme sprigs. Add the Worcestershire sauce and pepper. Serve hot.

PER SERVING: Calories: 314 | Protein: 18 g | Carbohydrates: 28 g | Fat: 14.9 g | Saturated Fat: 4.6 g | Cholesterol: 37 mg | Sodium: 189 mg | Potassium: 1000 mg | Phosphorus: 240 mg | Calcium: 73 mg | Fiber: 5 g | Exchanges: 1½ Starch, 1 Vegetable, 2 Lean Meat, 1½ Fat | Gluten Free: Use gluten-free flour, broth, and Worcestershire sauce

Gazpacho Mary

This is a chilled soup with the flavors of tomatoes, celery, and horseradish, like a puréed virgin Bloody Mary. It will enhance your daily intake of fiber exponentially and delectably.

INGREDIENTS | SERVES 4

3 large tomatoes
5 celery hearts
½ large yellow bell pepper
3 tablespoons shallot
½ medium cucumber
¼ cup lemon juice
4 teaspoons extra-virgin olive oil
¾ cup low-sodium tomato juice
½ teaspoon cayenne pepper sauce
1 teaspoon Worcestershire sauce
1 tablespoon grated horseradish
1 teaspoon garlic powder
½ teaspoon black pepper

Celery Hearts

Celery hearts are the most tender part of the plant. They are the innermost stalks of the bunch. Usually you can buy them pre-cut, approximately 8–9" from the base.

1. Chop the tomatoes and place them in a blender. Chop up one celery heart and save the others for garnish. Add the chopped one to the blender.

2. Chop the pepper, shallot, and cucumber and add them to the blender.

3. Add the remaining ingredients to the blender and purée until smooth and there are no large chunks.

4. Pour into glass tumblers and garnish with celery hearts. Serve chilled.

PER SERVING: Calories: 108 | Protein: 3 g | Carbohydrates: 15 g | Fat: 5.1 g | Saturated Fat: 0.7 g | Cholesterol: 0 mg | Sodium: 99 mg | Potassium: 715 mg | Phosphorus: 77 mg | Calcium: 58 mg | Fiber: 4 g | Exchanges: 3 Vegetable, 1 Fat or 1 Carbohydrate, 1 Fat | Gluten Free: Use gluten-free Worcestershire sauce

Pumpkin and Ginger Soup

Other types of winter squash may be substituted for the pumpkin.

INGREDIENTS | SERVES 4

1 tablespoon canola or grapeseed oil

1 medium-sized sweet onion, sliced

1 large stalk celery, sliced

2 bay leaves

¼ teaspoon dried thyme

¼ teaspoon dried oregano

4 medium carrots, sliced

2 cups pumpkin, cut into 1" cubes

3 tablespoons minced fresh ginger

4 cups water

½ teaspoon cinnamon

Pinch each of ground cloves, allspice, and mace (optional)

Freshly ground black pepper, to taste (optional)

Flavor Enhancing 101

A tablespoon of dry white wine or vermouth per serving is an excellent, low-sodium way to punch up the flavor of soup. Just be sure to add it to the soup during the cooking process to allow enough time for the alcohol to evaporate.

1. In a large saucepan, heat the oil and sauté the onions and celery, stirring until the onions are transparent, about 5–10 minutes.

2. Add the bay leaves, thyme, oregano, carrots, pumpkin, ginger, and water and bring to a boil. Reduce heat, cover, and simmer until the vegetables are tender, about 25 minutes.

3. Remove and discard the bay leaves. Use a hand blender to purée the soup. Alternatively, transfer the soup to a blender or food processor to purée it.

4. Serve warm, sprinkled with cinnamon, optional spices, and freshly ground black pepper, if desired.

PER SERVING: Calories: 102 | Protein: 2 g | Carbohydrates: 17 g | Fat: 3.8 g | Saturated Fat: 0.3 g | Cholesterol: 0 mg | Sodium: 70 mg | Potassium: 545 mg | Phosphorus: 74 mg | Calcium: 69 mg | Fiber: 3 g | Exchanges: 1 Starch, ½ Fat | Gluten Free

Crab Chowder

To get the best flavor for your chowder, use fresh Dungeness or several blue crabs.

INGREDIENTS | SERVES 6

2 pounds fresh crabs or 12 ounces canned crabmeat

6 cups milk

1 bay leaf

1 pinch saffron

2 leeks

1 large stalk celery

2 small red potatoes

2 whole artichokes, cooked, or 2 artichoke hearts, canned or frozen

1 cup water

2 tablespoons lemon juice

1 pinch cayenne pepper

1. If using fresh crab, boil in water for 3–6 minutes, depending upon the size. Remove the meat with a nutcracker and cut into large dice.

2. Combine the milk, bay leaf, and saffron in a soup pot. Over medium heat, bring to a boil. Add the crab and cover. Take off heat, keeping it covered, and let it stand.

3. Finely dice the white part of the leeks, the celery, and the potatoes. Remove the leaves and the center choke from the artichoke and dice the bottom (the heart).

4. In a saucepan, melt the butter and add all the vegetables, water, and lemon juice. Bring to a boil, reduce heat to medium, cover the pan, and cook for 10 minutes.

5. Take the cover off, turn the heat up, and cook until the liquids have evaporated. Turn the heat down to the lowest setting.

6. Add the crab and milk mixture along with the cayenne. Stir and warm thoroughly but slowly.

PER SERVING: Calories: 246 | Protein: 23 g | Carbohydrates: 32 g | Fat: 3.3 g | Saturated Fat: 1.8 g | Cholesterol: 63 mg | Sodium: 369 mg | Potassium: 1116 mg | Phosphorus: 475 mg | Calcium: 413 mg | Fiber: 5 g | Exchanges: ½ Starch, 1 Skim Milk, 2 Vegetable, 1½ Lean Meat | Gluten Free

Curried Zucchini Soup

*Five cups of chopped zucchini equals about 6 "baby" zucchinis,
2–3 medium sized ones, or 1 "jumbo" backyard garden variety.*

INGREDIENTS | SERVES 8

1 tablespoon olive oil

5 cups chopped zucchini

2 medium onions, chopped

1 medium celery stalk, diced

1 clove garlic, minced

2 teaspoons curry powder

¾ teaspoon salt

½ teaspoon cinnamon

¼ teaspoon pepper

1 teaspoon packed brown sugar

6 cups low-sodium vegetable or chicken broth

1. In a soup pot, heat the oil over medium heat and sauté the zucchini, onions, celery, garlic, curry powder, salt, cinnamon, and pepper, stirring occasionally, for about 10 minutes, until softened.

2. Sprinkle with the brown sugar and pour in the broth. Bring to a boil, then reduce to a simmer. Cook, covered, for 20 minutes, or until the vegetables are very tender.

3. In a blender or food processor, purée the soup in batches until smooth. Pour into a clean soup pot and reheat, but do not boil. Season with more salt and pepper, to taste.

PER SERVING: Calories: 72 | Protein: 5 g | Carbohydrates: 8 g | Fat: 3.0 g | Saturated Fat: 0.6 g | Cholesterol: 0 mg | Sodium: 285 mg | Potassium: 405 mg | Phosphorus: 93 mg | Calcium: 32 mg | Fiber: 2 g | Exchanges: 2 Vegetable, ½ Fat | Gluten Free: Use gluten-free broth

Tofu Soup with Rice

You can substitute bulgur, a crunchy, nutty wheat grain, for the rice in this recipe. However, bulgur is not gluten free.

INGREDIENTS | SERVES 8

6 cups low-sodium chicken, beef, or vegetable broth

6 cups mung bean sprouts

½ cup scallions

2 cups cilantro

2 tablespoons mint

1 cup fresh basil leaves

1 tablespoon chili oil or hot pepper sauce

Juice from 2 lemons

16 ounces firm tofu

4 cups cooked sticky white rice

1. Pour the broth into a large saucepan and heat on medium.

2. Mince the sprouts, scallions, cilantro, mint, and basil. In a bowl, toss them well with the chili oil and set aside to let the flavors mingle.

3. Juice the lemons and cut the tofu into 1" cubes.

4. Stir the lemon and tofu into the hot broth.

5. Place 1 cup of rice in the bottom of each serving bowl. Spoon the sprout and herb mixture on top of the rice and ladle the broth over the top.

PER SERVING: Calories: 179 | Protein: 12 g | Carbohydrates: 28 g | Fat: 3.0 g | Saturated Fat: 0.6 g | Cholesterol: 0 mg | Sodium: 87 mg | Potassium: 464 mg | Phosphorus: 161 mg | Calcium: 52 mg | Fiber: 3 g | Exchanges: 1½ Starch, 1 Vegetable, 1 Lean Meat | Gluten Free: Use gluten-free broth and tofu

Asian-Style Soup with Rice Noodles

This can be served in small bowls as a first course or in large bowls as lunch.
The contrast between soft and crunchy, spicy and sweet, makes this interesting.

INGREDIENTS | SERVES 4

1 quart low-sodium chicken broth

2 cloves garlic, minced

1" fresh ginger root, peeled and minced

1 cup scallions, thinly sliced

12 canned water chestnuts

1 cup bean sprouts, well rinsed

½ cup dry sherry

¼ cup low-sodium soy sauce

½ pound satin tofu

2 cups rice noodles, cooked

12 snow peas, sliced on the diagonal, for garnish

1. Bring the chicken broth to a boil and add all but the tofu, noodles, and snow peas. Cover and simmer for 10 minutes.

2. Add the tofu. Stir gently, then add the cooked noodles. Garnish with the snow peas, and serve.

PER SERVING: Calories: 228 | Protein: 11 g | Carbohydrates: 35 g | Fat: 3.3 g | Saturated Fat: 0.7 g | Cholesterol: 0 mg | Sodium: 700 mg | Potassium: 564 mg | Phosphorus: 187 mg | Calcium: 66 mg | Fiber: 3 g | Exchanges: 2 Starch, 1 Vegetable, 1 Lean Meat | Gluten Free: Use gluten-free broth, soy sauce, and tofu

Soy Galore

Tofu is made of soy and is related to all soy products, such as soy sauce, soy nuts, and soy paste. All are excellent food supplements. Tofu comes in satin (very soft and custardy), medium, and firm. The firm is excellent fried. A health benefit of tofu is that it has no cholesterol. Beware of soy sauce, however; it has approximately 1000 mg of sodium per tablespoon. Reduced- or low-salt soy sauce has approximately half of that.

CHAPTER 10

Meats and Poultry

Texas Burgers

You can make these burgers as spicy or as mild as you like.
Just make sure you use sugar-free chili sauce or you'll sweeten them up much too much.

INGREDIENTS | SERVES 4

1 pound lean ground sirloin
1 teaspoon garlic powder
1 tablespoon chili powder
½ cup red onion, minced
2 tablespoons sugar-free chili sauce
4 (6" diameter) grilled corn tortillas

1. Mix all ingredients but tortillas together. Form into patties.

2. Grill over medium-high flame or under the broiler to desired state of doneness.

3. Serve each burger on a grilled corn tortilla.

PER SERVING: Calories: 178 | Protein: 20 g | Carbohydrates: 14 g | Fat: 4.6 g | Saturated Fat: 1.4 g | Cholesterol: 52 mg | Sodium: 181 mg | Potassium: 439 mg | Phosphorus: 255 mg | Calcium: 51 mg | Fiber: 2 g | Exchanges: 1 Starch, 2½ Lean Meat | Gluten Free: Use gluten-free chili sauce

Pork Lo Mein

Chicken may be substituted for pork in this delectable recipe.

INGREDIENTS | SERVES 4

1½ tablespoons reduced-sodium soy sauce

1 teaspoon fresh ginger, grated

1 tablespoon rice vinegar

¼ teaspoon turmeric

¾ pound lean pork loin, cut into 1" cubes

½ cup green onion, sliced

2 teaspoons garlic, minced

2 cups cabbage, shredded

1 cup snap peas, cut into 1" pieces

½ tablespoon canola oil

¼ teaspoon crushed red pepper

2 cups whole-grain spaghetti, cooked

1 teaspoon sesame oil

1 teaspoon sesame seeds

1. Combine soy sauce, ginger, rice vinegar, and turmeric in a bowl. Mix in cubed pork and set aside.

2. Cut up onion, garlic, cabbage, and snap peas before starting stir-fry.

3. In large skillet or wok, heat oil and sauté onion and garlic. Add meat and cook quickly until meat and onions are slightly browned.

4. Add in cabbage and snap peas and continue to stir-fry for another 3–4 minutes. Sprinkle in crushed red pepper.

5. When vegetables are crisp-tender, add cooked pasta, sesame oil, and sesame seeds. Toss lightly, and serve.

PER SERVING: Calories: 278 | Protein: 17 g | Carbohydrates: 24 g | Fat: 13.3 g | Saturated Fat: 3.8 g | Cholesterol: 43 mg | Sodium: 275 mg | Potassium: 391 mg | Phosphorus: 221 mg | Calcium: 63 mg | Fiber: 5 g | Exchanges: 1 Starch, 2 Lean Meat, 1½ Fat | Gluten Free: Use gluten-free spaghetti and soy sauce

Is There a Difference Between Raw and Cooked Meat for Exchanges?

In calculations, 4 ounces of raw meat are equal to 3 ounces of cooked meat. This has been accounted for in the recipe analysis.

Southwest Black Bean Burgers

Pinto beans may be substituted for black beans if preferred.

INGREDIENTS | SERVES 5

1 cup cooked black beans, no salt added, drained and rinsed if canned

¼ cup onion, chopped

1 teaspoon chili powder

1 teaspoon ground cumin

1 tablespoon fresh parsley, minced

1 sprig fresh cilantro, minced

½ teaspoon salt

¾ pound 85% lean ground beef

Swapping Fresh Herbs for Dried

If you do not have fresh herbs such as parsley or cilantro available, 1 teaspoon dried may be used in place of 1 tablespoon fresh.

1. Place beans, onion, chili powder, cumin, parsley, cilantro, and salt in food processor. Combine ingredients using pulse setting until beans are partially puréed and all ingredients are mixed.

2. In a separate bowl, combine ground beef and bean mixture. Shape into 5 patties.

3. Meat mixture is quite soft after mixing and should be chilled or partially frozen prior to cooking. Grill or broil on oiled surface.

PER SERVING: Calories: 160 | Protein: 13 g | Carbohydrates: 10 g | Fat: 8 g | Saturated Fat: 3 g | Cholesterol: 34 mg | Sodium: 273 mg | Potassium: 305 mg | Phosphorus: 141 mg | Calcium: 25 mg | Fiber: 3.4 g | Exchanges: ½ Starch, 1½ Lean Meat, ½ Fat | Gluten Free

Asian Chicken Stir-Fry

Yellow summer squash is a thin-skinned squash like zucchini.
It has a mild, sweet flavor.

INGREDIENTS | SERVES 4

2 (5-ounce) boneless, skinless chicken breasts

½ cup low-sodium chicken broth

1 tablespoon low-sodium soy sauce

1 tablespoon cornstarch

1 tablespoon sherry

2 tablespoons peanut oil

1 medium onion, sliced

3 cloves garlic, minced

1 tablespoon grated ginger root

1 cup snow peas

½ cup canned sliced water chestnuts, drained

1 large yellow summer squash, sliced

¼ cup chopped dry-roasted unsalted peanuts

1. Cut chicken into strips and set aside. In small bowl, combine chicken broth, soy sauce, cornstarch, and sherry and set aside.

2. In large skillet or wok, heat peanut oil over medium-high heat. Add chicken and stir-fry until almost cooked, about 3–4 minutes. Remove to a plate.

3. Add onion, garlic, and ginger root to skillet and stir-fry for 4 minutes longer. Then add snow peas, water chestnuts, and squash and stir-fry for 2 minutes longer.

4. Stir chicken broth mixture and add to skillet along with chicken. Stir-fry for 3–4 minutes longer, or until chicken is thoroughly cooked and sauce is thickened and bubbly. Sprinkle with peanuts, and serve immediately.

PER SERVING: Calories: 232 | Protein: 16 g | Carbohydrates: 15 g | Fat: 13.2 g | Saturated Fat: 2.2 g | Cholesterol: 31 mg | Sodium: 320 mg | Potassium: 604 mg | Phosphorus: 242 mg | Calcium: 40 mg | Fiber: 3 g | Exchanges: 2 Lean Meat, 3 Vegetable, 1½ Fat | Gluten Free: Use gluten-free broth, soy sauce, and peanuts

Turkey Cutlets Florentine

The word "Florentine" on a menu means spinach.
This deep-green leaf is full of antioxidants and fiber, and it's delicious, too!

INGREDIENTS | SERVES 6

¼ cup water

½ cup dry breadcrumbs

½ teaspoon white pepper

2 tablespoons grated Parmesan cheese

6 (4-ounce) turkey cutlets

2 tablespoons olive oil

2 cloves minced garlic

2 (8-ounce) bags fresh baby spinach

¼ teaspoon ground nutmeg

⅓ cup shredded Jarlsberg cheese

Cheeses

You can use low-fat or nonfat cheeses, but they really don't have much flavor. Try using smaller amounts of very sharply flavored cheeses instead. Use extra-sharp Cheddar instead of Colby; Gruyère instead of Swiss; and Cotija instead of Parmesan. Grating or shredding cheese will also enhance the flavor and allow you to use less.

1. Pour water into a shallow bowl. On a shallow plate, combine breadcrumbs, pepper, and Parmesan and mix well.

2. Place turkey cutlets between waxed paper and pound to ⅛" thickness, if necessary. Dip cutlets into water, then into breadcrumb mixture to coat.

3. In a large saucepan, heat olive oil over medium-high heat. Add turkey cutlets and cook for 4 minutes. Carefully turn and cook for 4–6 minutes longer, until thoroughly cooked. Remove to serving plate and cover with foil to keep warm.

4. Add garlic to drippings remaining in pan and cook and stir for 1 minute.

5. Add spinach and nutmeg and cook and stir until spinach wilts, about 4–5 minutes.

6. Add the Jarlsberg, top with the turkey, cover, and remove from heat. Let stand for 2 minutes to melt cheese, then serve.

PER SERVING: Calories: 227 | Protein: 24 g | Carbohydrates: 10 g | Fat: 10.0 g | Saturated Fat: 3.0 g | Cholesterol: 62 mg | Sodium: 222 mg | Potassium: 702 mg | Phosphorus: 266 mg | Calcium: 171 mg | Fiber: 2g | Exchanges: ½ Starch, 1 Vegetable, 3 Lean Meat | Gluten Free: Use gluten-free bread crumbs

Turkey Breast with Dried Fruit

This is a good choice for smaller families celebrating Thanksgiving.
The sauce is delicious over mashed potatoes or steamed brown rice.

INGREDIENTS | SERVES 6

1½ pounds bone-in turkey breast

⅛ teaspoon salt

⅛ teaspoon pepper

1 tablespoon flour

1 tablespoon olive oil

1 tablespoon plant sterol margarine

½ cup pitted chopped prunes

½ cup chopped dried apricots

2 medium Granny Smith apples, peeled and chopped

1 cup low-sodium chicken broth

¼ cup Madeira wine

1. Sprinkle turkey with salt, pepper, and flour. In a large saucepan, heat olive oil and margarine over medium heat. Add turkey and cook until browned, about 5 minutes. Turn turkey.

2. Add all fruit to saucepan along with broth and wine. Cover and bring to a simmer. Reduce heat to medium low and simmer for 55–65 minutes, or until turkey is thoroughly cooked. Serve turkey with fruit and sauce.

PER SERVING: Calories: 296 | Protein: 21 g | Carbohydrates: 31 g | Fat: 9.6 g | Saturated Fat: 2.2 g | Cholesterol: 55 mg | Sodium: 129 mg | Potassium: 702 mg | Phosphorus: 211 mg | Calcium: 32 mg | Fiber: 3 g | Exchanges: 2 Fruit, 3 Lean Meat | Gluten Free: Use gluten-free flour, margarine, and broth

Keep the Skin

Keeping the skin on chicken and turkey while it's baking ensures the flesh will be moist and doesn't transfer much fat to the flesh. Just remove the skin and discard after cooking. The poultry will be much more flavorful and tender, and the fat content will be virtually the same as skinless.

Beef and Pumpkin Quinoa Pilaf

This hearty pilaf is delicious for a cold winter evening.
Serve it with a spinach salad and some breadsticks.

INGREDIENTS | SERVES 6

1 tablespoon olive oil

1 pound lean sirloin steak, cubed

1 medium onion, chopped

1 cup quinoa

2½ cups low-sodium beef broth

1 cup canned solid-pack pumpkin (no salt)

¼ cup grated Parmesan cheese

½ cup chopped flat-leaf parsley

1 tablespoon ground sage

½ teaspoon nutmeg

½ cup toasted no-salt pumpkin seeds

Pumpkins

Pumpkins are excellent sources of beta-carotene, vitamin C, and potassium. They can also help fight arteriosclerosis, or hardening of the arteries, which can lead to heart attacks. Pumpkin seeds are also a good source of zinc and unsaturated fatty acids.

1. In a large saucepan, heat olive oil over medium heat. Add steak and cook and stir until browned, about 5 minutes.

2. Add onion and cook and stir for 3 minutes longer. Add quinoa and stir.

3. Pour in the beef broth and bring to a simmer. Cover and simmer for 10 minutes.

4. Add pumpkin and cook and stir until hot, about 4 minutes.

5. Stir in Parmesan, parsley, sage leaves, and nutmeg. Pour into serving dish, and top with pumpkin seeds. Serve immediately.

PER SERVING: Calories: 307 | Protein: 22 g | Carbohydrates: 28 g | Fat: 12.2 g | Saturated Fat: 2.2 g | Cholesterol: 33 mg | Sodium: 135 mg | Potassium: 626 mg | Phosphorus: 333 mg | Calcium: 98 mg | Fiber: 5 g | Exchanges: 2 Starch, 2 Lean Meat, 1 Fat | Gluten Free: Use gluten-free broth

Pork Tenderloin with Blackberry Gastrique

This grilled pork tenderloin is glazed with whole-grain mustard and served with a tangy blackberry sauce. Serve it with delicious brown rice or couscous to sop up the flavors with healthy fiber. Garnish the roast with fresh mint leaves. (Couscous is not gluten free.)

INGREDIENTS | SERVES 6

1 tablespoon olive oil
1 tablespoon coarse-grain mustard
1½ pound pork tenderloin
1 teaspoon kosher salt
1 teaspoon ground black pepper
4 tablespoons minced shallot
½ cup blackberries, fresh or frozen
1 tablespoon balsamic vinegar
½ cup low-calorie blackberry preserves

Temperature Tip

The internal temperature of the tenderloin will go up about 5 degrees after it has been removed from the heat; it should be 155°F when done. The roast should be allowed to stand prior to cutting, covered with foil. This practice keeps the juices in the meat and makes it more succulent. Cutting the meat instantly makes the juices run out, leaving the meat dry.

1. Preheat a grill or grill pan over high heat.

2. Rub 1 teaspoon olive oil and coarse-grain mustard on the tenderloin, then sprinkle the kosher salt and black pepper on it.

3. Grill the tenderloin on all sides, for a total of about 10 minutes. Set the tenderloin aside, cover it with foil, and let it rest at least 10 minutes before slicing.

4. Sauté the shallots until tender in remaining olive oil. Remove from heat and stir in the blackberries, balsamic vinegar, and blackberry preserves.

5. Cut the tenderloin in ½"-thick slices, arrange the slices on a platter, and spoon the blackberry sauce over them.

PER SERVING: Calories: 158 | Protein: 22 g | Carbohydrates: 4 g | Fat: 5.3 g | Saturated Fat: 1.1 g | Cholesterol: 66 mg | Sodium: 560 mg | Potassium: 492 mg | Phosphorus: 268 mg | Calcium: 22 mg | Fiber: 2 g | Exchanges: 3 Lean Meat | Gluten Free

X Crunchy Oven-Fried Chicken Thighs

Oven frying is a lower-fat version of cooking compared to deep frying chicken.

INGREDIENTS | SERVES 4

4 small chicken thighs, skin removed

1 tablespoon unbleached all-purpose flour

1 large egg white

¼ teaspoon sea salt

½ teaspoon olive oil

1 tablespoon rice flour

1 tablespoon cornflake crumbs

Sack the Sodium

You can reduce the sodium in Crunchy Oven-Fried Chicken Thighs to 85.31 mg by omitting the salt and substituting an herb blend like Mrs. Dash Table Blend, the Spice House's Mr. Spice House Salt-Free Blend, or the Spice Hunter All-Purpose Chef's Blend.

1. Preheat oven to 350°F.

2. Rinse and dry the chicken thighs.

3. Put the flour on a plate.

4. In a small, shallow bowl, whip the egg white together with the sea salt. Add the olive oil and mix it into the egg white.

5. Put the rice flour and cornflake crumbs on another plate and mix them together.

6. Roll each chicken thigh in the flour, then dip it into the egg-white mixture, then roll it in the cornflakes crumbs mixture.

7. Place a rack on a baking sheet and spray with nonstick cooking spray. Arrange the chicken thighs on the rack so that they aren't touching. Bake for 35–45 minutes, until the meat juices run clear. (Note: If not using a rack, drain the thighs on paper towels to remove the excess fat before serving.)

PER SERVING: Calories: 88 | Protein: 11 g | Carbohydrates: 4 g | Fat: 2.6 g | Saturated Fat: 0.6 g | Cholesterol: 43 mg | Sodium: 207 mg | Potassium: 137 mg | Phosphorus: 93 mg | Calcium: 6 mg | Fiber: 0g | Exchanges: 1½ Lean Meat | Gluten Free: Use gluten-free flour and cornflake crumbs

Turkey Chili

If you like your chili spicy, do not remove the seeds from the jalapeño chilies.
This chili is delicious topped with grated Cheddar cheese.

INGREDIENTS | SERVES 6

1 pound uncooked turkey breast

½ medium onion

2 cloves garlic

2 tablespoons chopped jalapeño chilies

16 ounces white beans (cooked without salt)

1 (15-ounce) can low-sodium chickpeas, drained

2 tablespoons olive oil

4 teaspoons ground cumin

1 teaspoon marjoram

½ pound ground turkey

4 cups low-sodium chicken broth

¼ cup pearl barley

Hot sauce, to taste

Salt and pepper, to taste

1. Cut the turkey into ½" cubes. Mince the onion and garlic. Seed and chop the jalapeños. Drain and rinse the beans.

2. In a soup pot, heat the oil. Sauté the onion and garlic on medium heat for 3 minutes.

3. Stir in the cumin and marjoram and cook for 30 seconds.

4. Add both kinds of turkey, sautéing them until browned slightly.

5. Pour in the broth and stir in the barley and the jalapeños. Bring to a boil, reduce to a simmer, and cook for 30 minutes.

6. Add the beans, a dash of hot sauce, and salt and pepper, to taste. Simmer for another 10 minutes.

PER SERVING: Calories: 375 | Protein: 34 g | Carbohydrates: 41 g | Fat: 9.2 g | Saturated Fat: 1.8 g | Cholesterol: 58 mg | Sodium: 181 mg | Potassium: 872 mg | Phosphorus: 326 mg | Calcium: 129 mg | Fiber: 11 g | Exchanges: 2½ Starch, 1 Vegetable, 3 Lean Meat | Gluten Free: Replace the pearl barley with rice. Use gluten-free broth and beans.

Beef Pot Roast with Winter Vegetables

Use a slow cooker for most of the cooking in this recipe.
Set it up in the morning, let it run all day, and when you get home, dinner is done!

INGREDIENTS | SERVES 8

2½-pound bottom round roast, well trimmed

Salt and freshly ground pepper, to taste

1 tablespoon unsalted margarine (80% fat)

1 medium whole onion, cut in chunks

2 cloves garlic

2 large carrots, peeled and chopped

4 parsnips, peeled and chopped

4 baby blue-nose turnips, peeled and chopped

1 cup celery tops, chopped

3 large Yukon Gold potatoes, peeled and quartered

4 teaspoons chili sauce

2 (13-ounce) cans unsalted all-natural beef broth

1 teaspoon no-calorie sweetener such as Splenda

1 tablespoon low-sodium soy sauce

1. Sprinkle the beef with salt and pepper, if desired. Melt the margarine in a frying pan or Dutch oven over high heat and brown the beef. Keep the beef in the Dutch oven or transfer it to a slow cooker. Scrape up the brown bits on the pan with a bit of water and add to the slow cooker.

2. Add remaining ingredients to the pot. Set the slow cooker or oven to very low and let cook for 7–8 hours.

3. Slice the meat and divide dish into serving bowls. This dish makes its own gravy.

PER SERVING: Calories: 342 | Protein: 29 g | Carbohydrates: 39 g | Fat: 8.1 g | Saturated Fat: 2.5 g | Cholesterol: 63 mg | Sodium: 244 mg | Potassium: 1376 mg | Phosphorus: 381 mg | Calcium: 65 mg | Fiber: 6 g | Exchanges: 2 Starch, 2 Vegetable, 2½ Lean Meat | Gluten Free: Use gluten-free margarine, chili sauce, broth, and soy sauce

Pot Roast Trivia

New Englanders are credited with the dish we know as pot roast. They cooked tough cuts of meat in water or broth to tenderize them and make them suitable for the dinner table. Winter vegetables were readily available and added extra flavor.

Spicy Beef-Stuffed Mushrooms

The mushrooms should be 2½" across. This is a great side dish or appetizer.
Served over salad greens, stuffed mushrooms make a fine lunch.

INGREDIENTS | SERVES 4

½ pound chopped sirloin

½ cup minced onion

2 cloves garlic, minced

1" ginger root, peeled and minced

1 tablespoon canola oil

1 tablespoon Worcestershire sauce

Salt and freshly ground black pepper, to taste (optional)

1 large egg, slightly beaten

12–16 large mushroom caps, stems removed, brushed off

1. Sauté the meat, onion, garlic, and ginger in the oil, mixing constantly to break up lumps. When the meat turns pink (but not gray or brown), remove from the heat and add the Worcestershire sauce. Add salt and pepper, if desired. When almost cool, blend in the egg.

2. Preheat the oven to 350°F. Divide the stuffing between the mushrooms in a baking pan. Pour enough water to come ¼" up the sides in the pan.

3. Bake the mushrooms for 25 minutes. You can sprinkle them with chopped fresh herbs of your choice when done.

PER SERVING: Calories: 139 | Protein: 14 g | Carbohydrates: 7 g | Fat: 7.0 g | Saturated Fat: 1.4 g | Cholesterol: 79 mg | Sodium: 49 mg | Potassium: 523 mg | Phosphorus: 202 mg | Calcium: 21 mg | Fiber: 1 g | Exchanges: 1 Vegetable, 2 Lean Meat | Gluten Free: Use gluten-free Worcestershire sauce

Baked Chicken

You can replace the cream of chicken soup with low-sodium chicken broth if you prefer.

INGREDIENTS | SERVES 4

4 (4-ounce) boneless, skinless chicken breasts

1 (10¾-ounce) can reduced-sodium cream of chicken soup

½ cup low-fat shredded Swiss cheese

Go Nuts!

Crush pecans and sprinkle them over the chicken alone or with the shredded cheese for an extra crunch. Try more exotic nuts in your poultry dishes. Gingko nuts, the fruit of the gingko biloba, are preserved in brine and sold at specialty stores. They make a soft, sweet addition to poultry dishes.

1. Preheat oven to 350°F.

2. Spray a baking pan with light cooking spray.

3. Arrange chicken in pan.

4. Pour in chicken soup and 1 can of water.

5. Cover with foil and bake for 30 minutes.

6. Uncover chicken and sprinkle with Swiss cheese.

7. Bake for an extra 15 minutes.

PER SERVING: Calories: 188 | Protein: 25 g | Carbohydrates: 10 g | Fat: 4.8 g | Saturated Fat: 1.8 g | Cholesterol: 68 mg | Sodium: 428 mg | Potassium: 594 mg | Phosphorus: 330 mg | Calcium: 215 mg | Fiber: 0 g | Exchanges: ½ Starch, 3½ Lean Meat | Gluten Free: Use gluten-free soup and cheese

Smoked Turkey with Sour Apples

This is excellent for an after-school snack. It'll hold the kids over until dinner but not fill them up with a lot of simple sugars. Add Cheddar cheese if you want more substance.

INGREDIENTS | SERVES 4

1 tart green apple, peeled, cored, and cut in eighths
Juice of ½ lemon
8 slices deli smoked turkey

1. Core the apple and slice it into 8 pieces. Sprinkle with lemon juice.

2. Wrap each piece of apple in a smoked turkey slice. Use toothpicks if needed, and serve.

PER SERVING: Calories: 65 | Protein: 9 g | Carbohydrates: 7 g | Fat: 0.4 g | Saturated Fat: 0.1 g | Cholesterol: 19 mg | Sodium: 531 mg | Potassium: 145 mg | Phosphorus: 140 mg | Calcium: 7 mg | Fiber: 0g | Exchanges: ½ Fruit, 1 Lean Meat | Gluten Free

Chicken Thighs Cacciatore

For a nonalcoholic version, substitute red grape juice for the wine.

INGREDIENTS | SERVES 4

2 teaspoons olive oil

½ cup chopped onion

2 cloves garlic, minced

4 medium chicken thighs, skin removed

½ cup dry red wine

1 (14½-ounce) can unsalted diced tomatoes, undrained

1 teaspoon dried parsley

½ teaspoon dried oregano

¼ teaspoon pepper

⅛ teaspoon sugar

¼ cup grated Parmesan cheese

4 cups cooked spaghetti (no salt added in cooking)

2 teaspoons extra-virgin olive oil

For Red Wine Lovers

When a recipe calls for red wine, a dry red is usually preferable to sweeter wines. Dry wines are fermented until the natural sugars are gone. Types of dry red wines include Cabernet Sauvignon, Bordeaux, and Pinot Noir.

1. Heat a deep, nonstick skillet over medium-high heat and add the olive oil. Add the onion and sauté until transparent.

2. Add the garlic and chicken thighs and sauté for 3 minutes on each side, or until lightly browned. Remove thighs from the pan.

3. Add the wine, tomatoes and their juices, parsley, oregano, pepper, and sugar. Stir well, and bring to a boil.

4. Add the chicken back to the pan and sprinkle the Parmesan cheese over the top of the chicken and sauce. Cover, reduce heat, and simmer for 10 minutes. Uncover and simmer 10 more minutes.

5. To serve, put 1 cup of cooked pasta on each of 4 plates. Top each pasta serving with a chicken thigh and then divide the sauce between the dishes. Drizzle ½ teaspoon of extra-virgin olive oil over the top of each dish, and serve.

PER SERVING: Calories: 402 | Protein: 25 g | Carbohydrates: 45 g | Fat: 12.8 g | Saturated Fat: 3.4 g | Cholesterol: 55 mg | Sodium: 158 mg | Potassium: 430 mg | Phosphorus: 294 mg | Calcium: 141 mg | Fiber: 8 g | Exchanges: 3 Starch, 2 Lean Meat, 1 Fat | Gluten Free: Use gluten-free spaghetti

CHAPTER 11

Fish and Seafood

Poached Fish with Tomatoes and Capers

White fish fillets include cod, haddock, and pollock.
White fish is mild and sweet and cooks quickly.

INGREDIENTS | SERVES 4

2 tablespoons olive oil

½ cup chopped red onion

2 cloves garlic, minced

1 cup chopped fresh tomatoes

2 tablespoons no-salt tomato paste

¼ cup dry white wine

2 tablespoons capers, rinsed

4 (4-ounce) white fish fillets

¼ cup chopped parsley

1. In a large skillet, heat olive oil over medium heat. Add onion and garlic and cook and stir until tender, about 5 minutes.

2. Add tomatoes, tomato paste, and wine and bring to a simmer. Simmer for 5 minutes, stirring frequently.

3. Add capers to sauce and stir, then arrange fillets on top of sauce. Spoon sauce over fish. Reduce heat to low, cover, and poach for 7–10 minutes, or until fish flakes when tested with fork. Sprinkle with parsley, and serve immediately.

PER SERVING: Calories: 171 | Protein: 17 g | Carbohydrates: 6 g | Fat: 7.6 g | Saturated Fat: 1.1 g | Cholesterol: 49 mg | Sodium: 200 mg | Potassium: 523 mg | Phosphorus: 190 mg | Calcium: 51 mg | Fiber: 2 g | Exchanges: 1 Vegetable, 2 Lean Meat, ½ Fat (approximately 10 calories from alcohol are also included) | Gluten Free

Easy Oven-Roasted Salmon Steaks

Halibut steaks can be substituted for the salmon—its dense,
firm texture will hold up nicely while roasting.

INGREDIENTS | SERVES 4

4 (5-ounce) salmon fillets, skin on
2 teaspoons extra-virgin olive oil
1 teaspoon lemon pepper seasoning

Sodium Slashers

Fresh is usually best, but it isn't always practical. When it comes to seafood, frozen varieties are often frozen in a salty solution (brine). However, even fresh fish may be soaked in brine or sprayed with some other type of preservative to lengthen the shelf life. That's why it's important to wash off the fish using cold, unsoftened water.

1. Preheat oven to 350°F.

2. Rub ½ teaspoon of the olive oil into the flesh side of each salmon fillet. Sprinkle the lemon pepper over the olive oil-treated flesh and press it into the fish.

3. Treat an oven-safe baking dish with nonstick spray. Place the fillets skin-side down in the dish. Roast for 25 minutes.

PER SERVING: Calories: 146 | Protein: 19 g | Carbohydrates: 0 g | Fat: 7.4 g | Saturated Fat: 1.4 g | Cholesterol: 38 mg | Sodium: 58 mg | Potassium: 366 mg | Phosphorus: 224 mg | Calcium: 32 mg | Fiber: 0 g | Exchanges: 2½ Lean Meat | Gluten Free

Baked Red Snapper Almandine

Pecans may be substituted for the almonds for a unique twist,
but then you could not call it Almandine!

INGREDIENTS | SERVES 4

1 pound red snapper fillets

¼ teaspoon sea or kosher salt

Ground white or black pepper, to taste
(optional)

4 teaspoons all-purpose flour

2 teaspoons olive oil

2 tablespoons ground raw almonds

2 teaspoons unsalted tub margarine

1 tablespoon lemon juice

Red Snapper

Red snappers live in the Gulf of Mexico and
in the southeast Atlantic Ocean from North
Carolina to the Florida Keys. They are an
excellent source of protein and low in
sodium and saturated fat.

1. Preheat oven to 375°F. Rinse the red snapper fillets
   and dry between layers of paper towels. Season with
   salt and pepper, if using. Sprinkle the fillets with the
   flour, front and back.

2. In an ovenproof nonstick skillet, sauté the fillets in the
   olive oil until they are nicely browned on both sides,
   about 20 minutes.

3. Combine the ground almonds and margarine in a
   microwave-safe dish and microwave on high for 30
   seconds, or until the margarine is melted, then stir to
   combine.

4. Pour the almond-margarine mixture and the lemon
   juice over the fillets. Bake for 3–5 minutes, or until the
   almonds are nicely browned.

PER SERVING: Calories: 134 | Protein: 18 g | Carbohydrates: 3 g |
Fat: 5.3 g | Saturated Fat: 0.1 g | Cholesterol: 32 mg | Sodium:
202 mg | Potassium: 362 mg | Phosphorus: 172 mg | Calcium: 28 mg |
Fiber: 0.1 g | Exchanges 2½ Lean Meats | Gluten Free: Use gluten-
free flour and margarine

Fish Tacos

This is a fun recipe to serve at parties, and is easily doubled or tripled to feed a crowd. Get creative with your toppings—cheese, salsa, or diced bell pepper would all be delicious additions!

INGREDIENTS | SERVES 4

¼ cup light mayonnaise

½ cup plain nonfat yogurt

¼ cup onion, chopped

2 tablespoons jalapeño pepper, minced

1 sprig cilantro, minced

2 cups cabbage, shredded

¼ cup lime juice

1 clove garlic, minced

1 tablespoon canola oil

1 pound tilapia fillets

4 (6" diameter) corn tortillas

1 cup tomato, chopped

An Interesting Fact about Tortillas

For the same size tortilla, a corn tortilla is usually about half the calories as a wheat tortilla. Check labels in the store to compare.

1. In a medium bowl, whisk together mayonnaise, yogurt, onion, jalapeño, and cilantro. Stir in shredded cabbage and chill.

2. In a separate bowl, combine lime juice, garlic, and canola oil to make a marinade for fish. Pour over fish and cover and refrigerate at least 1 hour.

3. Place fish on aluminum foil-lined grill (spray foil with cooking spray) and cook 6–7 minutes on each side, until fish is tender and beginning to flake.

4. While fish is cooking, loosely wrap corn tortillas in large piece of aluminum foil to heat.

5. To assemble tacos, cut fish into strips and divide into 4 portions. Place strips in center of each heated tortilla. Top with coleslaw mixture and chopped tomatoes.

PER SERVING: Calories: 240 | Protein: 17 g | Carbohydrates: 22 g | Fat: 10.5 g | Saturated Fat: 1.7 g | Cholesterol: 38 mg | Sodium: 180 mg | Potassium: 556 mg | Phosphorus: 268 mg | Calcium: 117 mg | Fiber: 4 g | Exchanges: 1 Starch, 1 Vegetable, 2 Lean Meat, ½ Fat | Gluten Free: Use gluten-free mayonnaise and corn tortillas

Seared Scallops with Fruit

Serve this super quick and colorful dish with brown-rice pilaf and a green salad.

INGREDIENTS | SERVES 4

1 pound sea scallops

Dash salt

⅛ teaspoon white pepper

1 tablespoon olive oil

1 tablespoon unsalted tub margarine (80% fat)

2 medium peaches, sliced

¼ cup dry white wine

1 cup fresh blueberries

1 tablespoon lime juice

Scallops

Scallops are shellfish that are very low in fat. Sea scallops are the largest, followed by bay scallops and calico scallops. They should smell very fresh and slightly briny, like the sea. If they smell fishy, do not buy them. There may be a small muscle attached to the side of each scallop; pull that off and discard it because it can be tough.

1. Rinse scallops and pat dry. Sprinkle with salt and pepper and set aside.

2. In large skillet, heat olive oil and margarine over medium-high heat. Add the scallops and don't move them for 3 minutes. Carefully check to see if the scallops are deep golden brown. If they are, turn and cook for 1–2 minutes on the second side.

3. Remove scallops to serving plate. Add peaches to skillet and brown quickly on one side, about 2 minutes.

4. Turn the peaches, add wine to the skillet, and bring to a boil.

5. Remove from heat and add blueberries. Pour over scallops, sprinkle with lime juice, and serve immediately.

PER SERVING: Calories: 249 | Protein: 15 g | Carbohydrates: 15 g | Fat: 13.4 g | Saturated Fat: 2.0 g | Cholesterol: 28 mg | Sodium: 179 mg | Potassium: 461 mg | Phosphorus: 210 mg | Calcium: 30 mg | Fiber: 2 g | Exchanges: 1 Fruit, 2 Lean Meat, 1½ Fat (approximately 10 calories from alcohol are also included) | Gluten Free: Use gluten-free margarine

Sesame-Pepper Salmon Kabobs

Serve these skewers on brown-rice pilaf with a wedge of lemon on the side.
A fruit salad will round out the meal.

INGREDIENTS | SERVES 4

1 (1-pound) salmon steak
2 tablespoons olive oil, divided
¼ cup sesame seeds
1 teaspoon pepper
1 medium red bell pepper
1 large yellow bell pepper
1 medium red onion
8 cremini mushrooms
½ teaspoon salt

Can I Substitute Other Mushrooms for a Cremini Mushrooms?

Button mushrooms, cremini mushrooms, and portobello mushrooms are the same mushroom grown to different stages. The button mushroom is youngest, with the least flavor. As the mushroom matures, the flavor gets stronger. Portobellos are a bit stronger than creminis. Baby portobellos are actually cremini mushrooms. You may substitute other mushrooms, but the flavor will change.

1. Prepare and preheat grill. Cut salmon steak into 1" pieces, discarding skin and bones. Brush salmon with half of the olive oil.

2. In a small bowl, combine sesame seeds and pepper and mix. Press all sides of salmon cubes into the sesame seed mixture.

3. Slice bell peppers into 1" slices and cut red onion into 8 wedges. Trim mushroom stems and leave caps whole. Skewer coated salmon pieces, peppers, onion, and mushrooms on metal skewers. Brush vegetables with remaining olive oil and sprinkle with salt.

4. Grill 6" from medium coals, turning once during cooking time, until the sesame seeds are very brown and toasted and fish is just done, about 6–8 minutes. Serve immediately.

PER SERVING: Calories: 277 | Protein: 21 g | Carbohydrates: 12 g | Fat: 16.9 g | Saturated Fat: 2.4 g | Cholesterol: 47 mg | Sodium: 338 mg | Potassium: 842 mg | Phosphorus: 318 mg | Calcium: 46 mg | Fiber: 4 g | Exchanges: 2 Vegetable, 2½ Lean Meat, 2 Fat | Gluten Free

Curried Shrimp Salad in a Papaya

Chilled shrimp and toasted almonds complement the fruits and vegetables in this knockout luncheon salad. You can add some toasted sesame seeds to increase the nutrition and fiber value.

INGREDIENTS | SERVES 2

1 tablespoon olive oil

¼ cup plain nonfat yogurt

1 tablespoon lemon juice

1 teaspoon grated lemon zest

½ teaspoon curry powder

1 cup cooked peeled shrimp, chilled

¼ cup diced celery

¼ cup diced cucumber

10 seedless green grapes, halved

1 medium papaya

¼ cup unsalted dry roasted almonds, sliced

1. Whisk together olive oil, yogurt, lemon juice, lemon zest, and curry powder in a mixing bowl.

2. Add the shrimp, celery, cucumber, and grapes and toss to coat with the dressing. Chill salad until ready to serve.

3. Cut the papaya in half lengthwise through the stem area and scoop out the seeds.

4. Fill the papaya with the shrimp salad, mounding it up on top.

5. Sprinkle the almonds on top of the shrimp salad. Serve with a fork and spoon so the papaya flesh can be scooped and eaten after the salad is gone.

PER SERVING: Calories: 347 | Protein: 23 g | Carbohydrates: 28 g | Fat: 17.6 g | Saturated Fat: 2.0 g | Cholesterol: 119 mg | Sodium: 394 mg | Potassium: 824 mg | Phosphorus: 266 mg | Calcium: 196 mg | Fiber: 6 g | Exchanges: 1½ Fruit, ½ Vegetable, 3 Lean Meat, 2 Fat | Gluten Free

Grilled Mahi-Mahi with Pineapple Salsa

This salsa is also good on pork tenderloin.
The fruit and vegetables add fiber, texture, and piquancy to simple foods.

INGREDIENTS | SERVES 8

1 cup diced canned pineapple in juice, drained
½ cup diced red onion
¼ cup minced green bell pepper
¼ cup minced red bell pepper
¼ bunch cilantro
1 tablespoon white wine vinegar
¼ teaspoon hot pepper sauce
Salt, to taste (optional)
2 pounds mahi mahi or other firm-fleshed white fish
2 tablespoons olive oil
Pepper, to taste

1. Combine the pineapple, red onion, green bell pepper, and red bell pepper in a large bowl.

2. Chop the cilantro and add it to the bowl.

3. Add the vinegar, hot sauce, and a pinch of salt. Stir well, taste, and add more salt if needed.

4. Prepare your grill. Coat the fish with olive oil and season with pepper. Place on hot grill.

5. Cook for 3–4 minutes per side, or until fish is opaque. Top with pineapple salsa, and serve.

PER SERVING: Calories: 126 | Protein: 16 g | Carbohydrates: 7 g | Fat: 4.0 g | Saturated Fat: 0.6 g | Cholesterol: 37 mg | Sodium: 53 mg | Potassium: 441 mg | Phosphorus: 181 mg | Calcium: 23 mg | Fiber: 1 g | Exchanges: ½ Vegetable, 2 Lean Meat | Gluten Free: Use gluten-free hot pepper sauce

Baked Orange Roughy in White Wine

Catfish may be substituted for orange roughy for an interesting twist on this recipe.

INGREDIENTS | SERVES 4

4 (4-ounce) orange roughy fillets

2 tablespoons dry white wine

1 tablespoon lemon juice

1 teaspoon dried basil

½ teaspoon lemon zest

Freshly ground white or black pepper (optional)

Fishin' Down Under

Orange roughy lives in the deep cold waters off the coasts of New Zealand and Australia. If you have the choice, lighter meat is considered to be of higher quality.

1. Preheat oven to 425°F. Treat a baking dish with nonstick spray.

2. Rinse the fish fillets in cold water and pat dry.

3. Pour the wine and lemon juice into the prepared dish. Arrange the fillets in the dish, tucking under thin ends if necessary so the fillets are in an even layer.

4. Sprinkle the basil and lemon zest evenly over the fish. Season with pepper, if desired.

5. Cover the dish with foil. Bake until opaque through the thickest part, about 12–18 minutes, depending on the thickness of the fillets. Serve immediately.

PER SERVING: Calories: 67 | Protein: 14 g | Carbohydrates: 1 g | Fat: 0.6 g | Saturated Fat: 0 g | Cholesterol: 51 mg | Sodium: 62 mg | Potassium: 523 mg | Phosphorus: 159 mg | Calcium: 16 mg | Fiber: 0 g | Exchanges: 2 Lean Meat | Gluten Free

Baked Stuffed Shrimp

Serve one or two shrimp for an appetizer, four for lunch.
Make these easy and delicious stuffed shrimp ahead of time.

INGREDIENTS | SERVES 4

1 tablespoon unsalted tub margarine (80% fat)

2 cloves garlic, smashed

2 tablespoons Parmesan cheese

6 tablespoons bread crumbs

Juice of ½ lemon

1 teaspoon dried oregano

1 teaspoon freshly ground black pepper

16 extra-large to jumbo shrimp, peeled and butterflied

Fresh chopped parsley, for garnish

1. Preheat the oven to 500°F. Melt the margarine in a saucepan over medium heat. Sauté the garlic for about 4 minutes.

2. Stir in the next 5 ingredients and mix well.

3. Place the shrimp on a baking pan. Mound the stuffing on each.

4. Bake for about 6–8 minutes, or until the shrimp have turned pink and the stuffing is lightly browned. Garnish with parsley, and serve.

PER SERVING: Calories: 123 | Protein: 10 g | Carbohydrates: 9 g | Fat: 4.8 g | Saturated Fat: 1.2 g | Cholesterol: 60 mg | Sodium: 286 mg | Potassium: 98 mg | Phosphorus: 94 mg | Calcium: 78 mg | Fiber: 1 g | Exchanges: ½ Starch, 1 Lean Meat, ½ Fat | Gluten Free: Use gluten-free bread crumbs and margarine

Wild Versus Farm-Raised Shrimp

It was harder to get wild Gulf shrimp for months after the oil spill. However, the fishermen are back, so opt for wild shrimp if you can find them. They are more flavorful than their captivity-raised counterparts.

Lobster on the Grill

This is a lovely way to do lobster on the grill. The sauce is subtle enough, but adds a great flavor. Have your fishmonger split the lobster, removing the bitter parts of the head and the intestine.

INGREDIENTS | SERVES 2

½ cup red wine vinegar

1 tablespoon no-calorie sweetener such as Splenda

¼ cup freshly squeezed orange juice

Juice of ½ lemon

1 tablespoon olive oil

Salt and pepper, to taste

1 teaspoon fennel seeds

2 (1-pound) lobsters, split lengthwise in their shell

1. Bring the first 7 ingredients to a boil in a small saucepan. Reduce for 4 minutes. Meanwhile, heat the grill to medium or prepare your coals.

2. Brush sauce on the cut sides of the split lobster and place them on the grill, cut-side up. Close lid and let roast for 10 minutes, adding sauce every 5 minutes.

3. Turn and quickly grill cut-side down. Serve immediately, or chill and serve at a romantic picnic.

PER SERVING: Calories: 141 | Protein: 23 g | Carbohydrates: 7 g | Fat: 0.9 g | Saturated Fat: 0.1 g | Cholesterol: 78 mg | Sodium: 419 mg | Potassium: 499 mg | Phosphorus: 216 mg | Calcium: 86 mg | Fiber: 1 g | Exchanges: ½ Fruit, 3 Lean Meat | Gluten Free

Lobster Is a Treat

Its deliciousness makes lobster a treat, but it's very expensive. A 1-pound lobster provides approximately three-fourths of a cup of meat. Some people love the tails, while others eat nothing but the claws. The claws are very tender and sweet, and the tail meat is easier to get to and eat daintily. When it comes to a celebration, lobster cannot be beat!

Mexican-Style Corn Tortillas
Stuffed with Shrimp and Avocado

This is a fine lunch or brunch dish on a hot day, and especially good with margaritas or Bloody Marys.

INGREDIENTS | SERVES 6

6 (6" diameter) corn tortillas

24 large shrimp, peeled and deveined

½ cup dry white wine

6 medium California avocados, peeled and sliced

1 medium red onion, thinly sliced

Juice of 2 fresh limes

1 teaspoon freshly ground coriander seeds

1 tablespoon dried red pepper flakes

1 cup fresh or jarred salsa

6 ounces reduced-fat sour cream

½ cup chopped cilantro or parsley

Homemade Tortillas

You can make regular corn tortillas—the only hard part is getting them to be thin and crisp as opposed to thick and hard to eat. Serious Latin cooks buy a press to stamp out their tortillas.

1. Toast the tortillas and place on serving plates.

2. Poach the cleaned shrimp in the white wine and drain.

3. Stack 4 shrimp on each tortilla, add the avocado and onion, and sprinkle with lime juice, coriander, and pepper flakes.

4. Spoon salsa over each tortilla, add sour cream, and garnish with either cilantro or parsley.

PER SERVING: Calories: 275 | Protein: 11 g | Carbohydrates: 23 g | Fat: 15.8 g | Saturated Fat: 4.1 g | Cholesterol: 53 mg | Sodium: 265 mg | Potassium: 643 mg | Phosphorus: 202 mg | Calcium: 117 mg | Fiber: 7 g | Exchanges: 1 Starch, 1½ Vegetable, 1 Lean Meat, 2½ Fat (approximately 10 calories from alcohol are also included) | Gluten Free: Use gluten-free salsa and sour cream

Linguine with Shrimp

Throw this together for a quick family or company meal. It's just as good as it is easy.
Try it with artichokes or sun-dried tomatoes for extra sugar-free flavor.

INGREDIENTS | SERVES 10

1 pound shrimp, cooked

1 tablespoon olive oil

1 quart low-sodium garlicky tomato sauce

½ cup fresh Italian flat-leaf parsley, chopped

1 pound linguine, cooked without salt

1 teaspoon fresh lemon zest

1. Toss the shrimp in the oil over medium heat for 2 minutes.

2. Add the sauce and parsley. Cook for 5 minutes.

3. Add the linguine to the shrimp sauce. Sprinkle with lemon zest, and serve immediately.

PER SERVING: Calories: 276 | Protein: 20 g | Carbohydrates: 42 g | Fat: 3.4 g | Saturated Fat: 0.5 g | Cholesterol: 93 mg | Sodium: 294 mg | Potassium: 532 mg | Phosphorus: 190 mg | Calcium: 57 mg | Fiber: 3 g | Exchanges: 3 Starch, 1½ Lean Meat | Gluten Free: Use gluten-free linguine and tomato sauce

Baked Breaded Fish with Lemon

If French bread is not available, try using rolls.
The final dish will be just as delicious.

INGREDIENTS | SERVES 6

4 (1-ounce) slices French bread (stale, if possible)

1 teaspoon dried marjoram

1 teaspoon dried oregano

1 teaspoon dried sage

¼ teaspoon freshly ground white or black pepper

2 large lemons

1½ pounds halibut fillets

Canola spray oil with butter flavor

Things Could Get Steamy . . .

Steamers are a convenient way to prepare moist, healthy seafood. Because it circulates the air faster, the Cuisinart Turbo Convection Steamer cooks foods 33 percent faster than conventional models or bamboo steamers. You can use it to prepare an entire meal, and unlike conventional steaming methods, you don't have to rearrange or stir the foods during the steaming process.

1. Preheat the oven to 375°F. Treat a baking dish with nonstick spray.

2. Add the bread, seasoning, and pepper to the bowl of a food processor or a blender and process to mix and create bread crumbs. Set aside.

3. Wash the lemons and cut 1 into thin slices. Arrange the slices in the bottom of the prepared dish.

4. Grate the zest from the second lemon, then cut it in half and squeeze the juice into a shallow dish. Combine the grated zest with the prepared bread crumbs; set aside.

5. Rinse the fish fillets in cold water and pat dry with paper towels. Dip the fish pieces in the lemon juice and set them on the lemon slices in the baking dish.

6. Sprinkle the bread crumb mixture evenly over the fish pieces. Lightly mist the bread crumbs with the spray oil.

7. Bake until the crumbs are lightly browned and the fish is opaque, about 10–15 minutes. Baking time will depend on the thickness of the fish. Serve immediately, using the lemon slices as garnish.

PER SERVING: Calories: 219 | Protein: 15 g | Carbohydrates: 13 g | Fat: 12 g | Saturated Fat: 2 g | Cholesterol: 39 mg | Sodium: 191 mg | Potassium: 283 mg | Phosphorus: 163 mg | Calcium: 23 mg | Fiber: 1 g | Exchanges: ½ Starch, ½ Fruit, 2 Lean Meat, 1 Fat | Gluten Free: Use gluten-free bread

CHAPTER 12

Pasta, Rice, and Grains

Red Beans and Rice

A happy marriage of legume and grain, this is a Caribbean favorite that will fill up a family without leaving anyone hungry. You can substitute brown rice for extra fiber.

INGREDIENTS | SERVES 4

¼ cup diced celery

¼ cup diced onion

¼ cup diced green bell pepper

1 clove garlic, minced

1 tablespoon olive oil

¼ cup canned diced ham

2 cups red beans, cooked without salt

½ teaspoon dried thyme

¼ teaspoon cayenne pepper

¾ cup water

Salt, to taste

2 cups cooked white medium-grain rice

1. Sauté the celery, onion, green bell pepper, and garlic in olive oil.

2. Add the ham, beans, thyme, cayenne pepper, water, and salt.

3. Simmer for 45 minutes. Adjust seasonings, and serve over rice.

PER SERVING: Calories: 285 | Protein: 12 g | Carbohydrates: 48 g | Fat: 4.9 g | Saturated Fat: 0.9 g | Cholesterol: 3 mg | Sodium: 119 mg | Potassium: 480 mg | Phosphorus: 192 mg | Calcium: 73 mg | Fiber: 9 g | Exchanges: 3 Starch, 1 Vegetable, ½ Fat | Gluten Free

Whole-Wheat Couscous Salad

Couscous is semolina made from durum wheat,
and is one of the healthiest grain-based products.

1 cup low-sodium chicken broth

¼ cup dried currants

½ teaspoon cumin

¾ cup whole-wheat couscous

¼ cup olive oil

2 tablespoons lemon juice

1 cup broccoli, chopped and steamed crisp-tender

3 tablespoons pine nuts

1 tablespoon fresh parsley, chopped

1. Combine the chicken broth, currants, and cumin and bring to a boil.

2. Remove from heat and stir in the couscous. Cover and let sit until cool. Fluff couscous with fork 2–3 times during the cooling process.

3. Whisk together the olive oil and lemon juice.

4. Add the steamed broccoli and pine nuts to the couscous. Pour the oil and lemon juice over the couscous and toss lightly. Garnish with chopped parsley.

PER SERVING: Calories: 164 | Protein: 4 g | Carbohydrates: 18 g | Fat: 9.2 g | Saturated Fat: 1.2 g | Cholesterol: 0 mg | Sodium: 16 mg | Potassium: 156 mg | Phosphorus: 69 mg | Calcium: 17 mg | Fiber: 2 g | Exchanges: ½ Starch, 2 Vegetable, 1½ Fat | Gluten Free: This recipe is not gluten free

Aren't Currants Just Small Raisins?

Dried currants may look like a miniature raisin, but are actually quite different. Currants are berries from a shrub, not a vine, and there are red and black varieties. Black currants are rich in phytonutrients and antioxidants. They have twice the potassium of bananas and four times the vitamin C of oranges!

Beef Risotto

This elegant recipe is perfect for a spring dinner.
It is a last-minute recipe, so don't start it until after your guests have arrived.

INGREDIENTS | SERVES 6

2 cups water

2 cups low-sodium beef broth

2 tablespoons olive oil

½ pound sirloin steak, chopped

1 medium onion, minced

2 cloves garlic, minced

1½ cups arborio rice

2 tablespoons steak sauce

¼ teaspoon pepper

1 pound asparagus, cut into 2" pieces

¼ cup grated Parmesan cheese

2 teaspoons unsalted margarine (80% fat)

1. In a medium saucepan, combine the water and broth and heat over low heat until warm. Keep it on the heat.

2. In a large saucepan, heat olive oil over medium heat. Add the beef and cook and stir until browned. Remove it from the pan with a slotted spoon and set aside.

3. Add the onion and garlic to the pan and cook and stir until crisp-tender, about 4 minutes.

4. Add the rice and cook and stir for 2 minutes. Add the broth mixture, 1 cup at a time, stirring until the liquid is absorbed, about 15 minutes.

5. When there is 1 cup of broth remaining, return the beef to the pot and add the steak sauce, pepper, and asparagus. Cook and stir until the rice is tender, beef is cooked, and asparagus is tender, about 5 minutes. Stir in the Parmesan and margarine, and serve immediately.

PER SERVING: Calories: 333 | Protein: 15 g | Carbohydrates: 44 g | Fat: 10.1 g | Saturated Fat: 2.7 g | Cholesterol: 18 mg | Sodium: 169 mg | Potassium: 427 mg | Phosphorus: 198 mg | Calcium: 86 mg | Fiber: 3 g | Exchanges: 2½ Starch, 1½ Vegetable, 1 Lean Meat, 1 Fat | Gluten Free: Use gluten-free broth, steak sauce, and margarine

Farro Pilaf

You could substitute spelt or quinoa for the farro to omit the soaking step.
Just cook the grains in water until tender, according to package directions.

INGREDIENTS | SERVES 6

1½ cups farro
1 tablespoons plus 1 teaspoon olive oil
1 medium onion, chopped
4 cloves garlic, minced
1 cup shredded carrots
¼ cup dry white wine
⅛ teaspoon salt
⅛ teaspoon pepper

Farro

Farro is an ancient grain, cultivated by the Egyptians. It is wheat's ancestor. The dark grains, shaped like rice, have a nutty flavor and chewy texture. It must be soaked before cooking, so plan to make any recipe using farro ahead of time. The grain is full of fiber, protein, vitamins, and minerals.

1. Wash the farro well, picking out any foreign objects like chaff. Place in a large saucepan, add cold water to cover, and soak for 8 hours at room temperature.

2. Place the saucepan over high heat and bring to a boil. Reduce heat to low and simmer farro for 1½–2 hours, until tender but still chewy. Drain if necessary.

3. In another large saucepan, heat the olive oil over medium heat. Add the onion and garlic and cook and stir until crisp-tender, about 4 minutes.

4. Add carrots, then stir in cooked and drained farro. Cook and stir for 2–3 minutes.

5. Add wine, salt, and pepper and bring to a simmer. Simmer for 4–5 minutes, or until the wine is mostly absorbed. Stir, and serve immediately.

PER SERVING: Calories: 200 | Protein: 7 g | Carbohydrates: 35 g | Fat: 4.1 g | Saturated Fat: 0.6 g | Cholesterol: 0 mg | Sodium: 68 mg | Potassium: 279 mg | Phosphorus: 192 mg | Calcium: 28 mg | Fiber: 6 g | Exchanges: 2 Starch, 1 Vegetable, ½ Lean Meat | Gluten Free: Substitute quinoa for the farro (do not use spelt)

Acorn Squash, Cranberries, and Wild Rice

This is a quick and easy vegetarian meal made entirely in the microwave. The microwave takes the time factor out of cooking the squash, which can take 45–60 minutes in a conventional oven.

INGREDIENTS | SERVES 4

2 (4" diameter) acorn squash, whole

1 cup cooked wild rice

1 tablespoon balsamic vinegar

½ cup roasted unsalted pecans, chopped

½ cup dried cranberries

4 teaspoons maple syrup

All American

The combination of wild rice and cranberries is as American as a dish can be! Both of these ingredients were originally cultivated by Native Americans, who introduced them to the colonists. The sweet yet tart flavor of the cranberries pairs well with the nutty flavor of the rice and gives you all the fiber you need.

1. Pierce the squash all over with a fork. Place squash on a paper towel in the microwave oven. Cook on high for 5 minutes, turn over, and cook for 10 more minutes. Let stand 5–10 minutes.

2. Meanwhile, combine the cooked wild rice, balsamic vinegar, pecans, and dried cranberries. Set aside.

3. Cut the squash in half, remove the seeds, and place cut-side up in a casserole dish.

4. Spoon the wild rice mixture into the hollowed-out squash. Cover and cook on high in the microwave for several minutes to heat through.

5. Drizzle maple syrup on top before serving.

PER SERVING: Calories: 289 | Protein: 5 g | Carbohydrates: 50 g | Fat: 11 g | Saturated Fat: 1.1 g | Cholesterol: 0 mg | Sodium: 10 mg | Potassium: 867 mg | Phosphorus: 150 mg | Calcium: 89 mg | Fiber: 6 g | Exchanges: 2 Starch, 1 Fruit, 1½ Fat | Gluten Free: Use gluten-free maple syrup

Hoppin' John

This dish, a type of pilaf, consists of black-eyed peas and long-grain rice and is traditionally served on New Year's Eve in the southern United States. The peas are considered a good luck charm.

INGREDIENTS | SERVES 8

1¼ cups dried black-eyed peas

3 cups water

1½ cups diced onion

½ cup diced canned ham

½ teaspoon dried thyme

¼ teaspoon cayenne pepper

1 bay leaf

Salt and pepper, to taste

1 tablespoon unsalted tub margarine (80% fat)

1 tablespoon bacon fat

1½ cups long-grain rice

2¾ cups chicken broth

½ teaspoon salt

2 tablespoons chopped parsley

1. Put the black-eyed peas in a large pot and cover them with water to 1" above the peas. Bring to a boil and boil for 1 minute. Remove from heat and let sit for 90 minutes.

2. Drain and rinse the peas and return them to the pot along with the water, onion, ham, thyme, cayenne pepper, and bay leaf. Simmer uncovered for 25 minutes. Drain the liquid from the pot and remove the bay leaf. Season pea mixture with salt and pepper and set aside.

3. Melt the margarine and bacon fat in a large ovenproof pot and sauté the rice in it for 1 minute. Add the chicken broth and salt and bring to a simmer.

4. Meanwhile, preheat the oven to 325°F.

5. Stir the simmering rice once, cover, and bake for 25 minutes. Uncover and add the pea mixture and parsley. Cover and return to the oven for 5 minutes.

6. Remove from oven, fluff with a fork, and lightly toss to mix the ingredients together. Cover and let sit for 10 minutes, then serve.

PER SERVING: Calories: 288 | Protein: 13 g | Carbohydrates: 46 g | Fat: 6.3 g | Saturated Fat: 1.8 g | Cholesterol: 5 mg | Sodium: 301 mg | Potassium: 586 mg | Phosphorus: 280 mg | Calcium: 44 mg | Fiber: 5 g | Exchanges: 3 Starch, ½ Lean Meat, ½ Fat | Gluten Free: Use gluten-free broth and margarine

Curried Couscous

Curry powder is not one spice but a mixture of spices. Many times it includes a mixture of turmeric, cumin, cinnamon, and coriander, and many include other spices as well. Ingredients may vary, so check if you have an allergy.

INGREDIENTS | SERVES 8

1 tablespoon unsalted tub margarine (80% fat)

1 teaspoon curry powder

1½ cups couscous

1½ cups boiling water

¼ cup plain nonfat yogurt

3 tablespoons extra-virgin olive oil

1 teaspoon white wine vinegar

¼ teaspoon ground turmeric

¼ teaspoon lemon zest

1 teaspoon freshly ground black pepper

½ cup diced carrots

½ cup minced fresh parsley

½ cup seedless raisins

¼ cup blanched, sliced almonds

2 large scallions, white and green parts thinly sliced

¼ cup diced red onion

1½ teaspoons sesame oil

Curry It Up

There's a big difference in taste between "raw" curry powder and that which has been toasted or sautéed. Sautéing curry powder boosts the flavors, releasing the natural aromatic oils in the spices.

1. In a small nonstick skillet, melt the margarine until sizzling, then add the curry powder. Stir for several minutes, being careful not to burn the mixture.

2. Place the couscous in a medium-sized bowl. Pour enough of the boiling water into the pan with the sautéed curry powder to mix the curry and water as well as rinse out the pan.

3. Pour that and the remaining boiling water over the couscous. Cover tightly and allow the couscous to sit for 5 minutes. Fluff with a fork.

4. Mix together the yogurt, olive oil, vinegar, turmeric, lemon zest, and pepper and pour over the fluffed couscous, and mix well.

5. Add the carrots, parsley, raisins, almonds, scallions, red onion, and sesame oil and mix well. Serve at room temperature.

PER SERVING: Calories: 258 | Protein: 6 g | Carbohydrates: 37 g | Fat: 10 g | Saturated Fat: 1.3 g | Cholesterol: 0 mg | Sodium: 21 mg | Potassium: 259 mg | Phosphorus: 109 mg | Calcium: 55 mg | Fiber: 3 g | Exchanges: 2 Starch, ½ Fruit, 1½ Fat | Gluten Free: This recipe is not gluten free

Stir-Fried Singapore Noodles

Vermicelli noodles are sometimes known as rice sticks or rice noodles.

INGREDIENTS | SERVES 8

¼ teaspoon freshly ground pepper

⅛ teaspoon Oriental mustard powder

¼ cup roasted red bell pepper, finely minced

1 teaspoon low-sodium soy sauce

8 ounces vermicelli rice noodles

¼ cup sesame oil, divided

1 tablespoon curry powder

1 teaspoon turmeric powder

½ teaspoon low-sodium chicken bouillon powder

½ cup plus 2 tablespoons water

1 small red or sweet onion, thinly sliced

3 cloves garlic, sliced

3 small shallots, sliced

½ cup broccoli florets

½ cup cauliflower florets

4 large carrots, peeled and shredded

1 cup thinly sliced napa cabbage

2 red chilies, or to taste, seeded and minced

1 large egg, beaten

1 teaspoon honey (optional)

4 scallions, white and light green parts only, thinly sliced

Hot and Mellow

To turn Stir-Fried Singapore Noodles into a vegetarian main dish, you can substitute vegetable or mushroom broth for the chicken broth. Another way to turn this into a vegetarian dish and mellow the hotness of the chili is to use ½ cup apple juice for the liquid.

1. Add the pepper, mustard powder, bell pepper, and soy sauce to a small bowl and use a fork to mash and mix well. Set aside. Place noodles in lukewarm water to cover. Soak until soft, about 20 minutes. Drain.

2. Heat 2 tablespoons oil in a small nonstick sauté pan over medium heat. Add the curry and turmeric and cook for 1–2 minutes, or until fragrant. Add the chicken base and stir to dissolve. Add the red pepper mixture and ½ cup water and mix well. Remove from heat and set aside.

3. In a wok or large, deep nonstick sauté pan, heat the remaining oil over medium-high heat. Add the onions, garlic, and shallots and stir-fry until just wilted, about 1–2 minutes, stirring constantly.

4. Add the broccoli and cauliflower and stir-fry for 1 minute. Add 2 tablespoons water and stir. Add the carrots, cabbage, and chilies and cook until al dente, about 2 minutes. Push the vegetables to the side to make a well. Add the egg. Scramble until almost set, then incorporate into the other ingredients.

5. Push the vegetables to the side and add the red pepper mixture. Bring to temperature, then mix thoroughly. Taste; if hotter than you prefer, add the honey to mellow the flavor. Add the noodles and toss to combine. Cook to heat through. Stir in the scallions. Serve immediately.

PER SERVING: Calories: 287 | Protein: 5 g | Carbohydrates: 44 g | Fat: 10.7 g | Saturated Fat: 1.7 g | Cholesterol: 35 mg | Sodium: 194 mg | Potassium: 433 mg | Phosphorus: 134 mg | Calcium: 72 mg | Fiber: 4 g | Exchanges: 2½ Starch, 1 Vegetable, 1½ Fat | Gluten Free: Use gluten-free soy sauce, noodles, and bouillon powder

Toasted Walnut and Parsley Pesto with Noodles

Pesto is an Italian sauce usually made with oil, herbs, garlic, and cheese.

INGREDIENTS | SERVES 6

4 tablespoons chopped walnuts

4 tablespoons walnut oil

¾ cup fresh parsley

2 tablespoons grated Parmesan cheese

1 clove garlic, crushed

2 teaspoons fresh lemon juice

4 cups cooked egg noodles (cooked without salt)

Freshly ground black pepper, to taste

Seasoning Suggestions

Mrs. Dash Classic Italiano or Tomato Basil Garlic Seasoning Blend is good sprinkled over Italian dishes. You may also have some low-sodium seasoning blends to try.

1. In a small nonstick saucepan over medium heat, toast the walnuts until they're light brown, about 5–8 minutes, being careful not to burn them. Set aside to cool.

2. Add the oil, parsley, Parmesan, garlic, lemon juice, and half of the toasted walnuts to a food processor. Process until smooth.

3. In a large serving bowl, toss the noodles with the pesto and the remaining toasted walnuts. Grind the black pepper over the pasta, and serve.

PER SERVING: Calories: 281 | Protein: 7 g | Carbohydrates: 29 g | Fat: 16.1 g | Saturated Fat: 2.0 g | Cholesterol: 32 mg | Sodium: 36 mg | Potassium: 117 mg | Phosphorus: 121 mg | Calcium: 49 mg | Fiber: 2 g | Exchanges: 2 Starch, 3 Fat | Gluten Free: Use gluten-free noodles

Brown Rice with Bacon and Apples

You can serve this for breakfast, brunch, or as a side dish at dinner.

INGREDIENTS | SERVES 6

4 slices low-sodium pork bacon

1 tablespoon canola oil

1 cup sweet white onion, chopped

2 tart medium apples, peeled, cored, and chopped

½ cup jicama, peeled and diced

1 teaspoon freshly grated nutmeg

1 tablespoon no-calorie sweetener such as Splenda

3 cups brown rice, cooked without fat or salt

1. Cook the bacon until crisp. Crumble and set aside on a fresh paper towel. In a large frying pan, heat the oil over medium heat.

2. Sauté the onion for about 5 minutes.

3. Add the apples and jicama and stir. Mix in the rest of the ingredients.

PER SERVING: Calories: 179 | Protein: 4 g | Carbohydrates: 28 g | Fat: 5.8 g | Saturated Fat: 1.3 g | Cholesterol: 5 mg | Sodium: 57 mg | Potassium: 190 mg | Phosphorus: 92 mg | Calcium: 19 mg | Fiber: 3 g | Exchanges: 2 Starch, ½ Fat | Gluten Free: Use gluten-free bacon

Brown Rice

Brown rice has far more nutrition and flavor than white rice. White rice loses nutrients during processing, so brown rice contains more fiber and has more vitamin B per serving.

Indian Corn Cakes

Corn cakes are simple, delicious, and totally American!

Corn Lore

Native Americans saved early settlers in this country with their stores of corn. Native Americans taught the colonists how to grow, dry, and mill corn into meal. Corn as a crop started in ancient Mexico and Central America. The valuable crop went all the way to Canada, indicating tribal movement and sharing.

1. Bring the water to a boil and add salt.

2. Stir in the cornmeal and cook for about 20 minutes, stirring.

3. Add the pepper, molasses, and wild berries.

4. Prepare an 11" × 13" glass baking pan with nonstick spray. Spread the corn mixture in the pan and cover. Refrigerate for 1–2 hours, or until very stiff.

5. Heat margarine in a large frying pan. Cut the corn cakes into squares and fry until golden on both sides, approximately 5 minutes per side.

PER SERVING: Calories: 132 | Protein: 2.3 g | Carbohydrates: 19 g | Fat: 5.2 g | Saturated Fat: 1.0 g | Cholesterol: 0 mg | Sodium: 200 mg | Potassium: 95 mg | Phosphorus: 55 mg | Calcium: 9 mg | Fiber: 3 g | Exchanges: 1 Starch, 1 Fat | Gluten Free: Use gluten-free margarine

Tabouli Salad

This whole-grain salad is made from bulgur wheat, which is simply whole wheat berries that have been steamed, dried, cracked, and rehydrated. Much of the Middle East relies on various versions of tabouli to stretch its meat supply. It absorbs the flavors of spices, aromatic vegetables, and meats.

INGREDIENTS | SERVES 6

½ cup medium bulgur wheat
1½ cups water
⅓ cup lemon juice
2 tablespoons chopped fresh mint
1 teaspoon salt
1 teaspoon pepper
¼ cup extra-virgin olive oil
1 cup chopped fresh parsley
½ cup chopped green onions
2 large tomatoes, diced
1 tablespoon minced garlic

1. Soak the bulgur in the water for at least 2 hours.

2. Drain the excess water and put the bulgur in a large bowl.

3. Add the remaining ingredients to the bulgur and mix well.

4. Let sit at room temperature for 60 minutes, or refrigerate overnight.

5. Serve chilled, or at room temperature.

PER SERVING: Calories: 171 | Protein: 3 g | Carbohydrates: 18 g | Fat: 11 g | Saturated Fat: 1.5 g | Cholesterol: 0 mg | Sodium: 465 mg | Potassium: 312 mg | Phosphorus 71 mg | Calcium 41 mg | Fiber: 5 g | Exchanges: 1 Starch, 2 Fat | Gluten Free: This recipe cannot be made gluten free

Prepare Your Own Bulgur

If you soak 2 cups of wheat berries in 4 cups of water overnight, you can make your own bulgur the next day. Drain the wheat berries, simmer them in 4 cups of water for 60 minutes, and drain. Dry the wheat berries on a baking sheet pan in a 250°F oven for 45 minutes, or until dry. Chop up the dried, cooked wheat berries in a food processor and store in a large jar.

Asian Stir-Fried Rice

When cooking tofu, you need to press out the excess water, otherwise it splatters in hot oil and doesn't brown well. To do this, slice a block of tofu in half and wrap the cut pieces in layers of paper towels, changing the towels for new sheets when these get soaked. Some cooks suggest weighting the blocks of tofu down to press out more water.

INGREDIENTS | SERVES 4

2 tablespoons canola oil

8 ounces firm tofu, cubed

3 cloves garlic, crushed and minced

1 onion, diced

1 tablespoon minced fresh ginger, or to taste

1 cup cubed winter squash such as butternut or kabocha

1 cup shelled edamame

1 cup raw bamboo shoots

2 long green chilies, thinly sliced

2 cups cooked short-grain brown rice, chilled

3 tablespoons low-sodium soy sauce, or to taste

½ cup low-sodium vegetable broth or water, as needed

1. Heat the oil in a large wok or skillet over medium-high heat. Add and stir-fry the tofu, cooking it until it starts to brown, for 15–20 minutes. Remove it from the wok and set aside.

2. Add the garlic, onion, and ginger and stir-fry for about 1 minute.

3. Add the squash and edamame and stir-fry about 2 minutes.

4. Add the bamboo shoots, chilies, and rice, stirring well to combine. Add the soy sauce and cover the wok, cooking the mixture for about 5 minutes, or until the squash becomes tender. During the cooking, check that the mixture does not get too dry and add vegetable broth as needed, stirring it in well. Serve hot.

PER SERVING: Calories: 293 | Protein: 13 g | Carbohydrates: 39 g | Fat: 10.8 g | Saturated Fat: 1.0 g | Cholesterol: 0 mg | Sodium: 679 mg | Potassium: 863 mg | Phosphorus: 245 mg | Calcium 94 mg | Fiber: 5 g | Exchanges: 2½ Starch, 1 Lean Meat, 1 Fat | Gluten Free: Use gluten-free tofu, soy sauce, and broth

Why Chill the Rice?

If you don't chill cooked rice for stir-frying, the grains clump together and become mushy; also, it's likely they will absorb too much oil during the cooking. Stir-frying is a great way to use up leftover rice. This recipe calls for short-grain brown rice, which is somewhat sticky, but it provides a delicious texture and flavor for this dish. Any leftover rice will work.

CHAPTER 13

Beans and Lentils

✗ Spinach Salad with Navy Beans

You'll find dozens of recipes for spinach salads, but this particular dish has some unexpected flavors. Leftovers are great.

INGREDIENTS | SERVES 4

About 6 cups fresh baby spinach, well rinsed and dried

3 large hard-boiled eggs, quartered

2 cups navy beans, cooked from raw without salt

1 medium red onion, diced

½ cup soy bacon bits

½ cup toasted pumpkin seeds, without salt

1 thinly sliced jalapeño pepper

½ cup low fat, low calorie French salad dressing

Combine the spinach, eggs, beans, onion, soy bacon bits, pumpkin seeds, and jalapeño in a salad bowl. Dress as desired, and serve.

PER SERVING: Calories: 382 | Protein: 20 g | Carbohydrates: 46 g | Fat: 14.1 g | Saturated Fat: 2.5 g | Cholesterol: 159 mg | Sodium: 348 mg | Potassium: 835 mg | Phosphorus: 277 mg | Calcium 156 mg | Fiber: 14 g | Exchanges: 2 ½ Starch, 2 Vegetable, 1½ Lean Meat, 1 Fat | Gluten Free: Use gluten-free bacon bits and salad dressing

Edamame

*Edamame are fresh soybeans. They are the base of soy sauce, tofu, and soymilk.
You can eat them as a snack before sushi or as part of a crudités platter.
Edamame are also an excellent addition to salads, soups, and rice dishes.*

INGREDIENTS | SERVES 6

6 cups water
½ teaspoon salt
1 pound frozen edamame in pods

Snacks Should Be Healthful and Fun

Tastes are formed early. If your kids don't try something, don't make an issue, but keep presenting the food and see what happens. If you have a few kids in the house, have a "crunch contest"! Whose bite of celery or carrot or cucumber makes the loudest crunch? Everybody wins!

1. Bring the water and salt to a boil in a saucepan.

2. Add edamame and let the water come back to a boil.

3. Cook on medium-high for 5 minutes.

4. Drain the edamame, rinse with cold water, and drain again.

5. Serve either warm or cool.

PER SERVING: Calories: 83 | Protein: 8 g | Carbohydrates: 6 g | Fat: 3.6 g | Saturated Fat: 0 g | Cholesterol: 0 mg | Sodium: 205 mg | Potassium: 367 mg | Phosphorus: 122 mg | Calcium 53 mg | Fiber: 4 g | Exchanges: ½ Starch, 1 Lean Meat | Gluten Free

Minted Lentil and Tomato Salad

Different types of mint will change the flavor of this salad—so experiment, and enjoy!

INGREDIENTS | SERVES 6

1 cup dry lentils

2 cups water

½ cup onion, chopped

2 teaspoons garlic, minced

¼ cup celery, chopped

½ cup green pepper, chopped

½ cup parsley, finely chopped

2 tablespoons fresh mint, finely chopped, or 2 teaspoons dried

¼ cup lemon juice

¼ cup olive oil

½ teaspoon salt

1 cup fresh tomato, diced

1. Place the lentils and water in a medium-sized saucepan and bring to a quick boil. Reduce heat, cover, and cook on low 15–20 minutes, or until tender. Drain and transfer to a medium bowl.

2. Add the onion, garlic, celery, green pepper, parsley, and mint and mix well.

3. In a small bowl, whisk together the lemon juice, olive oil, and salt. Pour into lentils and mix well. Cover and refrigerate several hours.

4. Before serving, mix in diced tomato.

PER SERVING: Calories: 209 | Protein: 9 g | Carbohydrates: 23 g | Fat: 10 g | Saturated Fat: 1.4 g | Cholesterol: 0 mg | Sodium: 209 mg | Potassium: 354 mg | Phosphorus 114 mg | Calcium 36 mg | Fiber: 6 g | Exchange: 1½ Starch, ½ Lean Meat, 1½ Fat | Gluten Free

Chickpeas in Lettuce Wraps

Lettuce wraps are a low-calorie way to serve delicious individual portions.

INGREDIENTS | SERVES 8

1 (16-ounce) can unsalted chickpeas

3 tablespoons olive oil

3 tablespoons lemon juice

3 cloves garlic, minced

1 tablespoon chopped fresh mint

½ cup diced red onion

8 lettuce leaves

1 cup chopped tomatoes

1 cup chopped yellow bell pepper

Chickpeas

Chickpeas, also known as garbanzo beans, are a round legume with a nutty flavor and tender texture. One cup of cooked beans provides more than 10 grams of fiber. Eating high-fiber foods reduces cholesterol and helps prevent heart disease. The beans are also very high in folate, the molecule that reduces homocysteine levels.

1. Drain the chickpeas, rinse, and drain again. Place half in a blender or food processor. Add the olive oil, lemon juice, garlic, and mint and blend or process until smooth.

2. Place in a medium bowl and stir in the remaining chickpeas and red onion until combined.

3. To make sandwiches, place lettuce leaves on a work surface. Divide the chickpea mixture among the leaves and top with tomatoes and bell pepper. Roll up, folding in sides, to enclose filling. Serve immediately.

PER SERVING: Calories: 124 | Protein: 4 g | Carbohydrates: 14 g | Fat: 6.2 g | Saturated Fat: 0.8 g | Cholesterol: 0 mg | Sodium: 7 mg | Potassium: 253 mg | Phosphorus: 81 mg | Calcium: 32 mg | Fiber: 3 g | Exchanges: ½ Starch, 1½ Vegetable, 1 Fat | Gluten Free

Green Lentil Salad

Green lentils are smaller and plumper than other lentils, which makes them look like the caviar of lentils. The French have been making lentil salad for centuries. When you make it yourself, you can cook the lentils to your preference.

INGREDIENTS | SERVES 4

1 cup dried French green lentils

5 cups water

1 bay leaf

2 tablespoons olive oil

1 medium carrot, finely chopped

1 medium celery stalk, finely chopped

2 tablespoons minced shallots

1 teaspoon minced garlic

2 tablespoons extra-virgin olive oil

¼ cup lemon juice

1 teaspoon grated lemon zest

1 tablespoon chopped fresh thyme

1 tablespoon chopped fresh parsley

¼ teaspoon ground coriander

Salt and pepper, to taste

1. Put the lentils, water, and bay leaf in a saucepan. Bring to a boil, reduce heat, and simmer for 20 minutes. Drain in a colander, remove the bay leaf, and let the lentils cool. Put them in a large bowl and set aside.

2. Heat the olive oil in a sauté pan and cook the carrot, celery, and shallots over medium heat until tender, about 5 minutes. Add to the lentils.

3. Add the garlic, extra-virgin olive oil, lemon juice, lemon zest, thyme, parsley, coriander, salt, and pepper to the lentils. Toss to combine, and chill.

4. Serve chilled, or at room temperature.

PER SERVING: Calories: 306 | Protein: 13 g | Carbohydrates: 33 g | Fat: 14 g | Saturated Fat: 2.0 g | Cholesterol: 0 mg | Sodium: 35 mg | Potassium: 582 mg | Phosphorus: 12 mg | Calcium: 55 mg | Fiber: 16 g | Exchanges: 2 Starch, ½ Vegetable, 1 Lean Meat, 2 Fat | Gluten Free

Kidney Bean Chili

Garnish each individual serving with a few cooked corn kernels,
some grated Cheddar cheese, and a sprinkling of chopped cashews, if desired.

INGREDIENTS | SERVES 4

2 tablespoons canola oil

1 medium green bell pepper, chopped

1 medium celery stalk, chopped

1 small onion, chopped

1 medium carrot, shredded

1 medium zucchini, shredded

1 clove garlic, minced

1 (16-ounce) can low-sodium chopped tomatoes

1 (16-ounce) can cooked kidney beans

1 cup unsalted tomato sauce

¼ cup water

2 teaspoons chili powder

¼ teaspoon hot pepper sauce

1 teaspoon ground basil

1 teaspoon oregano

¾ teaspoon black pepper

¼ cup cooked corn kernels, shredded

1. In a large saucepan or soup pot, heat the oil. Sauté the green pepper, celery, onion, carrot, zucchini, and garlic on medium for 3 minutes.

2. Add all the remaining ingredients. Bring to a boil, reduce to a simmer, and cook for 5 more minutes.

PER SERVING: Calories: 268 | Protein: 10 g | Carbohydrates: 43 g | Fat: 8.3 g | Saturated Fat: 0.8 g | Cholesterol: 0 mg | Sodium: 364 mg | Potassium: 1167 mg | Phosphorus: 215 mg | Calcium: 129 mg | Fiber: 12 g | Exchanges: 2 Starch, 2 Vegetable, ½ Lean Meat, 1 Fat | Gluten Free: Use gluten-free tomato sauce and pepper sauce

Beans Count

You can soak beans overnight and then cook them, or buy them canned, without losing much of their nutritional makeup. However, canned beans can be very high in sodium. Look for no-sodium or reduced-sodium selections. Beans are a good substitute for animal proteins in vegetarian cooking, and they add to any meal, vegetarian or not.

Indian-Style Chicken with Lentils

In countries with huge populations, it's both wise and popular to stretch meat,
fish, and seafood with all kinds of legumes.

INGREDIENTS | SERVES 5

1 cup lentils

3 cups water

¼ teaspoon salt

¼ teaspoon red pepper flakes, or to taste

2 cloves garlic, peeled and minced

1 medium onion, peeled and finely minced

2 tablespoons lemon juice

1 teaspoon cumin

½ cup chopped fresh parsley

1 pound boneless, skinless chicken breasts, cut into bite-sized pieces

1 cup low-fat plain yogurt

1 tablespoon curry powder

¼ teaspoon salt, or to taste

¼ teaspoon Tabasco sauce, or to taste

1. Place the lentils and water in a saucepan. Bring to a boil, reduce heat, and simmer.

2. Just before the lentils are cooked (when barely tender, after about 25 minutes), add the salt, pepper flakes, garlic, onion, lemon juice, cumin, and parsley.

3. Toss the chicken with the yogurt, curry powder, salt, and Tabasco. Place on aluminum foil and broil for 5 minutes per side.

4. Mix the chicken into the lentils, and serve with rice.

PER SERVING: Calories: 262 | Protein: 28 g | Carbohydrates: 31 g | Fat: 3.3 g | Saturated Fat: 1.0 g | Cholesterol: 46 mg | Sodium: 358 mg | Potassium: 831 mg | Phosphorus: 400 mg | Calcium: 139 mg | Fiber: 13 g | Exchanges: 2 Starch, 3 Lean Meat | Gluten Free

Veggie-Stuffed Zucchini

Stuff the zucchini with any vegetables you like.
The vegetables in this recipe can easily be substituted with your favorites.

INGREDIENTS | YIELDS 4 SERVINGS

4 medium zucchini

1 teaspoon salt

2 teaspoons unsalted tub margarine (80% fat)

2 teaspoons canola oil

1 medium onion, chopped

1 clove garlic, crushed

½ cup unsalted cooked chickpeas

2 tablespoons flour

1 teaspoon ground coriander

1 large potato, peeled, cooked, and diced

1 cup frozen green peas, defrosted

2 tablespoons chopped cilantro

1. Preheat oven to 375°F.

2. Cut each zucchini in half lengthwise and scoop out the pulp. Place each half with the open side up on a shallow roasting pan and sprinkle with salt.

3. Heat margarine and oil in a skillet over medium heat. Add the onion and garlic and sauté for 4 minutes.

4. Stir in the chickpeas, flour, coriander, potato, green peas, and cilantro.

5. Spoon ¼ of the potato mixture into each zucchini half and cover it with foil.

6. Bake for 15 minutes, or until zucchini is tender.

PER SERVING: Calories: 238 | Protein: 9 g | Carbohydrates: 40 g | Fat: 5.6 g | Saturated Fat: 0.7 g | Cholesterol: 0 mg | Sodium: 635 mg | Potassium: 758 mg | Phosphorus: 185 mg | Calcium: 59 mg | Fiber: 7 g | Exchanges: 2 Starch, 1 Vegetable, 1 Fat | Gluten Free: Use gluten-free flour, margarine, and chickpeas

Vegan Recipes

Vegan recipes do not have animal products included in the ingredients. Look for margarines that do not contain whey or any dairy components.

Lentil Stew

Lentils cook up fast, but if you are in a big hurry, use canned lentils for convenience's sake. Offer this stew with slices of hot, buttery baguette, which you can spark with sprinkles of garlic powder, and a simple salad of lightly dressed greens.

INGREDIENTS | SERVES 4

2 tablespoons olive oil

1 large sweet onion, thinly sliced

5 cloves garlic, minced

2 cups cooked lentils without fat or salt

3 large tomatoes, quartered

2 large banana peppers, stemmed and quartered lengthwise

2 soy "sausage" patties, cut in small pieces

1 large portobello mushroom, thinly sliced

1 cup low-sodium vegetable or chicken broth

¼ teaspoon salt

Freshly ground black pepper, to taste

1. Heat the oil in a large skillet over medium heat and sauté the onion for 8–10 minutes, or until golden.

2. Add the garlic, lentils, tomatoes, peppers, "sausages," and mushroom, stirring well.

3. Reduce the heat to medium-low and continue cooking until the onions and peppers soften, about 10 minutes.

4. Add the vegetable broth as the mixture begins to dry out. Stir in the salt and pepper. Serve hot.

PER SERVING: Calories: 214 | Protein: 10 g | Carbohydrates: 27 g | Fat: 9.2 g | Saturated Fat: 1.2 g | Cholesterol: 0 mg | Sodium: 251mg | Potassium: 869 mg | Phosphorus: 217 mg | Calcium: 60 mg | Fiber: 8 g | Exchanges: 1½ Starch, 1 Vegetable, ½ Lean Meat, 1 Fat | Gluten Free: Use gluten-free soy sausage and broth

CHAPTER 14

Vegetables

Eggplant and Tomato Stew

*This vegetable stew is delicious garnished with a dollop of yogurt and a sprinkling of chopped parsley.
If you like a little spice, add hot pepper sauce.*

INGREDIENTS | SERVES 4

2 eggplants, trimmed but left whole

2 teaspoons olive oil

1 medium-sized Spanish onion, chopped

1 teaspoon chopped garlic

2 cups canned unsalted tomatoes, chopped, undrained

1. Preheat oven to 400°F.

2. Roast the eggplants on a baking sheet until soft, about 45 minutes. Remove all the meat from the eggplants.

3. In a large sauté pan, heat the oil and sauté the onions and garlic. Add the eggplant and tomatoes.

4. Remove from heat, transfer to a food processor, and pulse until it becomes creamy. Serve at room temperature.

PER SERVING: Calories: 107 | Protein: 4 g | Carbohydrates: 21 g | Fat: 2.9 g | Saturated Fat 0.4 g | Cholesterol: 0.0 mg | Sodium: 18 mg | Potassium: 795 mg | Phosphorus: 89 mg | Calcium: 65 mg | Fiber: 10 g | Exchanges: 4 Vegetable and ½ Fat; or 1 Carbohydrate, 1 Vegetable, and ½ Fat | Gluten Free

Indian Vegetable Cakes

This is a great way to get kids to eat their veggies!
A nonstick pan helps to prevent sticking. Sour cream makes a very good garnish.

INGREDIENTS | SERVES 6

1 tablespoon olive oil

1 (10-ounce) package frozen chopped spinach, thawed and squeezed of excess moisture

½ box (5 ounces) frozen baby peas, thawed

½ cup scallions, chopped

1 teaspoon curry powder

Salt and hot pepper sauce, to taste

¼ cup cornmeal

5 extra-large eggs, well beaten

½ cup Parmesan cheese

1. Heat olive oil in a nonstick pan over a medium flame.

2. Mix together all ingredients except Parmesan cheese.

3. Drop patties, 3 or 4 at a time, into the pan and fry until delicately browned, about 5 minutes per side. Turn, and sprinkle with cheese.

PER SERVING: Calories: 180 | Protein: 13 g | Carbohydrates: 11 g | Fat: 10 g | Saturated Fat 3.3 g | Cholesterol: 205 mg | Sodium: 255 mg | Potassium: 313 mg | Phosphorus: 217 mg | Calcium: 188 mg | Fiber: 3 g | Exchanges: ½ Starch, 1 Vegetable, 1 Lean Meat, 1½ Fat | Gluten Free: Use gluten-free frozen vegetables

Oven-Roasted Corn on the Cob

This is one of the easiest recipes you'll find, but it's oh so good!

INGREDIENTS | SERVES 4

4 medium ears fresh sweet corn
1 tablespoon fresh lime juice
Freshly ground black pepper, to taste

1. Preheat oven to 350°F.

2. Peel back the corn husks and remove any silk. Brush the corn with the lime juice and grind black pepper over the corn. Pull the husks back up over the corn, twisting the husks at the top to keep them sealed.

3. Place the corn on the rack in a roasting pan large enough to hold the ears without overlapping. Roast for 30 minutes, or until the corn is heated through and tender.

4. Peel back the husks and use them as a handle, if desired, or discard the husks and insert corn holders into the ends of the cobs. Serve immediately.

PER SERVING: Calories: 89 | Protein: 3 g | Carbohydrates: 19 g | Fat: 1.3 g | Saturated Fat: 0.3 g | Cholesterol: 0.0 mg | Sodium: 15 mg | Potassium: 280 mg | Phosphorus: 91 mg | Calcium: 3 mg | Fiber: 2 g | Exchanges: 1 Starch | Gluten Free

Caramelized Spiced Carrots

This is a simple side dish that is full of flavor.
Serve it with grilled or roasted chicken, or during the holidays along with a baked ham.

INGREDIENTS | SERVES 4

1¼ pounds baby carrots
¼ cup orange juice
⅛ teaspoon salt
⅛ teaspoon white pepper
1 teaspoon grated orange zest
1 tablespoon sugar
1 tablespoon grated ginger root
1 tablespoon plant sterol margarine

1. In a large saucepan, combine the carrots, orange juice, salt, and pepper. Bring to a boil over high heat, then reduce heat to low, cover, and cook for 3–4 minutes, or until carrots are crisp-tender.

2. Add the orange zest, sugar, ginger root, and margarine and bring to a boil over high heat. Cook until most of the orange juice evaporates and the carrots start to brown, stirring frequently, about 4–5 minutes. Serve immediately.

PER SERVING: Calories: 83 | Protein: 1 g | Carbohydrates: 17 g | Fat: 1.6 g | Saturated Fat 0.2g | Cholesterol: 0.0 mg | Sodium: 208 mg | Potassium: 375 mg | Phosphorus: 43 mg | Calcium: 51 mg | Fiber: 4 g | Exchanges: ½ Fruit, 2 Vegetable | Gluten Free: Use gluten-free margarine

Baby Carrots

Since appearing on the market not so very long ago, baby carrots have overtaken regular carrots in sales. They are not technically baby carrots, but a carrot variety called Imperator that is grown to be longer and sweeter than regular carrots. The carrots are then trimmed down to the baby carrot shape and size.

Veggie-Stuffed Tomatoes

This cold side dish can also be served as a vegetarian entrée along with a fruit salad and some breadsticks.

INGREDIENTS | SERVES 4

1 tablespoon olive oil

1 medium onion, chopped

3 cloves garlic, minced

1 medium green bell pepper, chopped

4 large celery stalks, chopped

1 tablespoon fresh chives, chopped

2 teaspoons fresh oregano leaves

⅛ teaspoon salt

⅛ teaspoon pepper

½ cup plain yogurt

1 tablespoon lime juice

2 tablespoons grated Parmesan cheese

4 large (3" diameter) tomatoes

1. In a medium saucepan, heat the olive oil over medium heat. Add the onion, garlic, and green bell pepper and cook and stir until crisp-tender, about 4 minutes.

2. Remove from heat and stir in the celery, chives, oregano, salt, and pepper. Remove to a medium bowl and chill until cold, about 1 hour.

3. Stir the yogurt, lime juice, and Parmesan into cooled vegetable mixture.

4. Cut the tops off the tomatoes and gently scoop out tomato flesh and seeds, leaving a ½" shell. Stuff with the vegetable mixture. Cover and chill for 2–3 hours before serving.

PER SERVING: Calories: 122 | Protein: 6 g | Carbohydrates: 17 g | Fat: 4.7 g | Saturated Fat: 1.0 g | Cholesterol: 3 mg | Sodium: 198 mg | Potassium: 788 mg | Phosphorus: 144 mg | Calcium: 148 mg | Fiber: 4 g | Exchanges: 3 Vegetable, 1 Fat | Gluten Free

Sesame Green Beans

Crunchy green beans and sesame are seasoned with sesame oil for this vegetarian side dish. Leftovers will stand up with a shot of lemon juice or vinegar.

INGREDIENTS | SERVES 4

1 pound fresh green beans
1 tablespoon sesame oil
½ teaspoon salt
¼ teaspoon pepper
¼ cup sesame seeds

Sesame Asparagus

Take a bunch of asparagus and trim about 2" off the bottom. Blanch them in boiling water and shock them in cold water like the green beans. Cut the asparagus on the diagonal into ½" pieces and sauté them in sesame oil. Season them and sprinkle with sesame seeds.

1. Trim the stem ends off the green beans.

2. Add the green beans to boiling water and cook them for 5 minutes.

3. Drain the beans and plunge them into ice water. Drain them again.

4. Heat a sauté pan over medium heat and add the sesame oil to it. Sauté the beans in the sesame oil for 3 minutes.

5. Season the beans with salt and pepper and sprinkle the sesame seeds over them. Serve hot.

PER SERVING: Calories: 119 | Protein: 4 g | Carbohydrates: 11 g | Fat: 8.0 g | Saturated Fat: 1.1 g | Cholesterol: 0.0 mg | Sodium: 301mg | Potassium: 276 mg | Phosphorus: 116 mg | Calcium: 55 mg | Fiber: 6 g | Exchanges: 2 Vegetable, 1½ Fat | Gluten Free

Grilled Mushroom and Vegetable Medley

Splash a zero calorie vinaigrette dressing over the vegetables before serving.

INGREDIENTS | SERVES 8

Canola spray oil with butter flavor

1 large red bell pepper, seeded and cut into ¼" strips

1 large green bell pepper, seeded and cut into ¼" strips

2 medium-size zucchini, sliced crosswise into ¼" slices

2 medium-size yellow squash, sliced crosswise into ¼" slices

2 cups fresh button mushrooms, sliced

4 medium-size green onions, white and green parts minced

1 teaspoon dried thyme

1 teaspoon dried basil

½ teaspoon garlic powder

¼ teaspoon mustard powder

⅛ teaspoon freshly ground black pepper

1. Prepare a 20" × 14" sheet of heavy-duty foil by spraying the center with a spray oil.

2. Arrange the vegetables over the foil. Evenly sprinkle the green onions, thyme, basil, garlic and mustard powders, and black pepper over the vegetables. Lightly spray the mixture with the spray oil. Fold the ends of the foil up and over the vegetables, wrapping it into a packet and sealing it by crimping the edges well, leaving space for heat to circulate.

3. Grill on a covered grill over medium coals for 20–25 minutes, or until the vegetables are fork tender. Carefully open the foil packet and grill for an additional 5 minutes to let the juices from the vegetables evaporate, if desired.

PER SERVING: Calories: 34 | Protein: 2 g | Carbohydrates: 7 g | Fat: 0.4 g | Saturated Fat: 0.1 g | Cholesterol: 0.0 mg | Sodium: 10 mg | Potassium: 423 mg | Phosphorus: 67 mg | Calcium: 32 mg | Fiber: 2 g | Exchanges: 1½ Vegetable | Gluten Free

X Sweet Potato Mash

Sweet potatoes originally come from Central and South America.
They make a delectable side dish for any occasion!

INGREDIENTS | SERVES 4

4 (5" diameter) sweet potatoes, peeled and cubed

2 teaspoons lemon juice

4 teaspoons unsalted tub margarine (80% fat)

¼ teaspoon ground cumin

¼ teaspoon ground cinnamon

¼ teaspoon dried ginger

¼ teaspoon chipotle powder or other salt-free chili powder (optional)

½ cup skim milk

1. In a saucepan, cover the sweet potatoes with cold water and add the lemon juice. Bring to a boil over medium heat, cover, and cook for 7–10 minutes, until the potatoes are fork tender. Once the sweet potatoes are fully cooked, drain the water from the pot and place them in a medium-sized bowl.

2. Melt the margarine in the saucepan over medium heat. Add the cumin, cinnamon, ginger, and chipotle powder, if desired, and sauté for 30 seconds. Add the milk and bring to a boil.

3. Pour over the cooked sweet potatoes. Mix together using a masher or wooden spoon. Serve immediately.

PER SERVING: Calories: 157 | Protein: 3 g | Carbohydrates: 28 g | Fat: 3.9 g | Saturated Fat: 0.7 g | Cholesterol: 1 mg | Sodium: 86 mg | Potassium: 490 mg | Phosphorus: 91 mg | Calcium: 78 mg | Fiber: 4 g | Exchanges: 2 Starch | Gluten Free: Use gluten-free margarine

X Vegetables in Warm Citrus Vinaigrette

You can substitute reduced fresh orange juice for the frozen fruit juice concentrate and water called for in this recipe. Using a frozen fruit juice concentrate saves some time, however, because you can simply mix it to the strength you need.

INGREDIENTS | SERVES 4

½ teaspoon saffron

¼ teaspoon lemon or lime zest

2 teaspoons grapeseed oil

1 tablespoon water

Grapeseed spray oil

1 (10-ounce) package frozen mixed vegetables (corn, lima beans, peas, green beans, and carrots), thawed

1 tablespoon orange juice concentrate

⅛ teaspoon freshly ground black pepper

1. Preheat oven to 350°F.

2. Add the saffron, zest, grapeseed oil, and water to a microwave-safe bowl. Microwave on high for 20–30 seconds, until the water just boils, then stir. Cover and set aside to infuse at room temperature while the vegetables bake.

3. Treat an ovenproof casserole dish with the spray oil and add the thawed vegetables. Spray a light coating of additional spray oil over the top of the vegetables. Cover and bake for 15 minutes. Carefully remove the cover and stir the vegetables. Spray with an additional coating of spray oil. Bake for an additional 15 minutes.

4. During the last few minutes of the baking time, add the frozen orange juice concentrate to the saffron-oil mixture. Whisk to combine.

5. Remove the vegetables from the oven. Pour the saffron-orange vinaigrette over the vegetables, add the pepper, and toss to combine. Serve immediately.

PER SERVING: Calories: 81 | Protein: 2 g | Carbohydrates: 11 g | Fat: 3.4 g | Saturated Fat: 0.5 g | Cholesterol: 0 mg | Sodium: 179 mg | Potassium: 143 mg | Phosphorus: 38 mg | Calcium: 20 mg | Fiber: 3 g | Exchanges: ½ Starch, 1 Vegetable, ½ Fat | Gluten Free

Herbed Dilled Lima Beans

Lima beans are thought to originate in Peru.
Remember your geography—Lima is the capital of Peru!

INGREDIENTS | SERVES 4

1 (10-ounce) package frozen lima beans, thawed

¾ cup apple cider vinegar

¾ cup water

¼ teaspoon cayenne pepper or dried red pepper flakes

2 cloves garlic, minced

2 teaspoons dill seeds

1 teaspoon dried dill weed

¼ teaspoon salt

1. Put the thawed lima beans in a glass jar or other covered container large enough to hold the beans and vinegar mixture.

2. In a medium nonreactive saucepan over high heat, bring the vinegar and water to a boil. Stir in the cayenne pepper, garlic, dill seeds and weed, and salt. Pour the vinegar mixture over the beans and allow to cool to room temperature.

3. Cover and refrigerate for 24 hours before serving.

PER SERVING: Calories: 108 | Protein: 5 g | Carbohydrates: 17 g | Fat: 1.7 g | Saturated Fat: 0.3 g | Cholesterol: 0 mg | Sodium: 369 mg | Potassium: 340 mg | Phosphorus: 92 mg | Calcium: 51 mg | Fiber: 5 g | Exchanges: 1¼ Startch/Gluten Free

Kohlrabi with Lemon

Kohlrabi is a very sweet and delicious vegetable available in the fall and winter.
It tastes wonderful sprinkled with grated Parmesan cheese and run under the broiler.

INGREDIENTS | SERVES 4

1 pound kohlrabi, stems removed, peeled, and sliced

½ cup low-sodium chicken broth

Juice of ½ lemon

Salt and pepper, to taste

½ cup fresh parsley, chopped

1. Place the kohlrabi slices in a saucepan.

2. Add the broth, lemon juice, salt, and pepper.

3. Simmer over low heat for 25–30 minutes. Sprinkle with parsley. Serve hot.

PER SERVING: Calories: 40 | Protein: 3 g | Carbohydrates: 8 g | Fat: 0.4 g | Saturated Fat: 0.1 g | Cholesterol: 0.0 mg | Sodium: 36 mg | Potassium: 472 mg | Phosphorus: 66 mg | Calcium: 39 mg | Fiber: 4 g | Exchanges: 1½ Vegetable | Gluten Free: Use gluten-free broth

Kohlrabi Tales

This name of this strange-sounding cruciferous vegetable comes from the German word *kohl* for "cabbage" and *rabi,* which means "turnip." Kohlrabi is a member of the family of cruciferous vegetables, which also includes Brussels sprouts, broccoli, and cabbage. Sometimes it is hard to find, but is a wonderful vegetable when you can!

Pumpkin Soufflé

This is a very good substitute for potatoes on a festive occasion.
It goes well with poultry and game.

INGREDIENTS | SERVES 4

1 (13-ounce) can unsalted puréed pumpkin
2 large egg yolks
½ cup half-and-half
2 tablespoons no-calorie sweetener such as Splenda
¼ teaspoon cloves
½ teaspoon cinnamon
¼ teaspoon nutmeg
¼ teaspoon allspice
½ teaspoon salt
1 teaspoon orange zest
5 egg whites, beaten stiff

1. Preheat the oven to 400°F. Prepare a soufflé dish with nonstick spray.

2. Put all ingredients but the egg whites in your electric mixer and beat until smooth.

3. Gently fold in the egg whites.

4. Scrape into the soufflé mold. Bake for 55 minutes.

5. Check for doneness by inserting a knife. If it comes out clean, the soufflé is done. Serve immediately.

PER SERVING: Calories: 123 | Protein: 8 g | Carbohydrates: 11 g | Fat: 6.2 g | Saturated Fat 3.2 g | Cholesterol: 116 mg | Sodium: 381 mg | Potassium: 311 mg | Phosphorus: 101 mg | Calcium: 76 mg | Fiber: 3 g | Exchanges: ½ Starch, 1 Lean Meat, ½ Fat | Gluten Free

Colcannon

The combination of cabbage and mashed potatoes is classic Irish fare.
Potatoes have long been a fibrous staple in the Irish diet.

INGREDIENTS | SERVES 6

1 pound kale

2 teaspoons olive oil

3 large potatoes, about 3 pounds

½ teaspoon kosher salt

2 tablespoons unsalted tub margarine (80% fat)

⅓ cup nonfat milk

½ teaspoon white pepper

1. Pull the stems off the kale and discard. Chop the greens and sauté them in olive oil over medium heat for 15 minutes. Take them off the heat and reserve.

2. Peel potatoes and cut them into 2" pieces. Put potato pieces in a pot with cold water to cover and salt.

3. Turn heat to medium-high and bring potatoes to a boil. Turn down to a simmer and cook until the potatoes can be easily pierced with a fork, about 15 minutes.

4. Drain the potatoes in a colander, then put them in a bowl and mash them with a potato masher, or put them through a ricer. Add margarine and milk and mix to a creamy consistency. Season with white pepper.

5. Add the sautéed kale to the mashed potatoes and fold it in. Serve hot.

PER SERVING: Calories: 265 | Protein: 8 g | Carbohydrates: 48 g | Fat: 6.0 g | Saturated Fat 1.0 g | Cholesterol: 0.0 mg | Sodium: 247 mg | Potassium: 1315 mg | Phosphorus: 186 mg | Calcium: 147 mg | Fiber: 5 g | Exchanges: 2½ Starch, 2 Vegetable, ½ Fat | Gluten Free: Use gluten-free margarine

Crunchy Sautéed New Potatoes

Just about everyone loves this recipe! It's quick to make and very tasty.
The potatoes get quite crisp as the water evaporates and cooks them through.
Add fresh parsley just before serving for extra color and kick.

INGREDIENTS | SERVES 4

2 tablespoons olive oil

2 tablespoons water

8 small-sized new or red potatoes, scrubbed and halved

Salt and pepper, to taste

1. Add the oil and water to a nonstick pan over medium heat.

2. Place the potatoes in the pan, cut-sides down. Cover and cook for 10 minutes.

3. Remove the lid and continue to brown until the cut sides are crisp. Turn, and sprinkle with salt and pepper, if desired.

PER SERVING: Calories: 296 | Protein: 8 g | Carbohydrates: 56 g | Fat: 7.2 g | Saturated Fat: 1.2 g | Cholesterol: 0.0 mg | Sodium: 20 mg | Potassium: 1548 mg | Phosphorus: 208 mg | Calcium: 36 mg | Fiber: 4 g | Exchanges: 2 Starch | Gluten Free

CHAPTER 15

Salads and Salad Dressings

Buttermilk Dressing

Buttermilk is naturally thick and tastes rich, even though it's low in fat.
This classic dressing is perfect drizzled over mixed greens.

INGREDIENTS | SERVES 4

¾ cup low-fat buttermilk

2 tablespoons low-fat or light mayonnaise

2 tablespoons lemon juice

2 medium shallots, chopped

⅛ teaspoon salt

1 tablespoon chopped chives

5 sprigs chopped fresh dill

⅛ teaspoon pepper

1. Combine all ingredients in blender or food processor and blend or process until mixed.

2. Cover, and store in refrigerator for up to 4 days.

PER SERVING: Calories: 47 | Protein: 2 g | Carbohydrates: 4 g | Fat: 3.0 g | Saturated Fat: 0.7 g | Cholesterol: 5 mg | Sodium: 174 mg | Potassium: 106 mg | Phosphorus: 48 mg | Calcium: 62 mg | Fiber: 0 g | Exchanges: ⅓ Skim Milk, ½ Fat | Gluten Free: Use gluten-free mayonnaise

Broccoli Slaw

Broccoli, carrots, raisins, and almonds provide lots of fiber and flavor in this salad. It's especially good for kids who won't eat cooked broccoli. You can give them this in place of a hot vegetable.

INGREDIENTS | SERVES 4

3 cups blanched broccoli florets

¼ cup shredded carrot

2 tablespoons mayonnaise

1 teaspoon Dijon mustard

1 tablespoon red wine vinegar

1 tablespoon minced shallots

¼ cup golden raisins

½ cup toasted sliced almonds

Salt and pepper, to taste

1. Mix all the ingredients together.

2. Refrigerate at least 60 minutes before serving.

PER SERVING: Calories: 185 | Protein: 6 g | Carbohydrates: 17 g | Fat: 12.0 g | Saturated Fat: 1.1 g | Cholesterol: 3 mg | Sodium: 91 mg | Potassium: 436 mg | Phosphorus: 147 mg | Calcium: 86 mg | Fiber: 4 g | Exchanges: 3 Vegetable, 2½ Fat | Gluten Free: Use gluten-free mayonnaise and mustard

Tofu, Oil, and Vinegar Salad Dressing

This salad dressing is very adaptable.
Try adding your choice of fresh or dried herbs, spices, or freshly ground black pepper.

INGREDIENTS | SERVES 4

1 tablespoon plus 1 teaspoon extra-virgin olive oil

2 tablespoons firm silken tofu

1 tablespoon cider vinegar

1 teaspoon ground mustard

1. Put all the ingredients in a small bowl and whisk to combine.

2. Pour over prepared salad greens and vegetables.

PER SERVING: Calories: 47 | Protein: 1 g | Carbohydrates: 0 g | Fat: 4.8 g | Saturated Fat: 0.7 g | Cholesterol: 0 mg | Sodium: 3 mg | Potassium: 19 mg | Phosphorus: 10 mg | Calcium: 4 mg | Fiber: 0 g | Exchanges: 1 Fat | Gluten Free: Use gluten free tofu and mustard

Chunky Chicken Salad

Use leftover chicken or buy precut chicken to save time.
If you want the low-sodium values of this recipe, make sure the chicken was cooked without seasonings.

INGREDIENTS | SERVES 6

1 pound cooked chicken breast, cut into 1" slices

1 cup finely diced celery

½ cup finely diced sweet onion

3 tablespoons sweet relish

½ cup low-fat mayonnaise

Salt and pepper, to taste

1. Combine all the ingredients in a salad bowl.

2. Cover, and refrigerate.

PER SERVING: Calories: 191 | Protein: 24 g | Carbohydrates: 8 g | Fat: 6.8 g | Saturated Fat: 1.5 g | Cholesterol: 69 mg | Sodium: 236 mg | Potassium: 269 mg | Phosphorus: 182 mg | Calcium: 23 mg | Fiber: 1 g | Exchanges: 1½ Vegetable, 3 Lean Meat | Gluten Free: Use gluten-free relish and mayonnaise

Fill Up on Salad

Lettuce and tomatoes can be very filling, especially when served with chicken salad. Hearty salads can replace meaty meals, a good way to ensure you get enough protein and vegetables. Tucking your salad in whole-wheat pita bread takes care of a serving of grains, as well.

Roasted Baby Beet Salad

This is a very pretty salad; the red of the beets contrasts with the white yogurt and green romaine leaves. You can garnish the salad with chopped toasted walnuts.

INGREDIENTS | SERVES 4

8 baby beets
2 tablespoons olive oil
2 tablespoons white wine vinegar
¼ teaspoon salt
⅛ teaspoon white pepper
½ teaspoon dried dill weed
4 cups torn romaine leaves
½ sweet onion, sliced
½ cup low-fat plain yogurt

Oh, Those Beets!

Beets are a wonderful, colorful vegetable that are low in calories and fat. They are commonly used in salads and soups. In Australia, they are even put on hamburgers.

1. Preheat oven to 350°F.

2. Wash the beets and scrub them gently. Cut off the stems and root ends. Wrap them in aluminum foil and place on a cookie sheet.

3. Roast for 30–40 minutes, or until tender. Let cool. Slip the beets from their skins and slice thinly.

4. In a small bowl, toss the beets with the oil and vinegar and sprinkle with salt, pepper, and dill.

5. In a large serving bowl, toss the beets with the romaine and onions. Spoon a dollop of yogurt on each salad, and serve immediately.

PER SERVING: Calories: 139 | Protein: 4 g | Carbohydrates: 15 g | Fat: 7.6 g | Saturated Fat: 1.3 g | Cholesterol: 2 mg | Sodium: 241 mg | Potassium: 523 mg | Phosphorus: 105 mg | Calcium: 96 mg | Fiber: 4 g | Exchanges: 3 Vegetable, 1½ Fat | Gluten Free

Cucumber-Mango Salad

The combination of cucumbers and mangoes is delicious and very fresh.
This salad is the ideal complement to grilled fish.

INGREDIENTS | SERVES 4

¾ cup plain low-fat yogurt

¼ cup low-fat buttermilk

2 tablespoons lemon juice

1 tablespoon honey

2 tablespoons chopped fresh dill

½ cup finely chopped red onion

2 medium cucumbers

3 cups ripe mango cubes

1. In a large bowl, combine the yogurt, buttermilk, lemon juice, honey, dill, and onion and mix well with a wire whisk.

2. Peel the cucumbers and cut them in half lengthwise. Using a spoon, scoop out the seeds. Cut them into ¼" slices and add to the yogurt mixture.

3. Peel mangoes and, standing them on end, slice down around the pit to remove the flesh. Cut them into cubes, add them to the yogurt mixture, and toss gently. Serve immediately, or chill for 2–3 hours before serving.

PER SERVING: Calories: 156 | Protein: 5 g | Carbohydrates: 34 g | Fat: 1.6 g | Saturated Fat: 0.8 g | Cholesterol: 4 mg | Sodium: 53 mg | Potassium: 506 mg | Phosphorus: 120 mg | Calcium: 138 mg | Fiber: 3 g | Exchanges: 1½ Fruit, ½ Skim Milk, 1 Vegetable | Gluten Free

Apple Coleslaw

Adding sweet and tart apples to a classic coleslaw is a delicious new twist.
Serve it with some grilled salmon for a fabulous meal.

INGREDIENTS | SERVES 8

1 cup plain nonfat yogurt

¼ cup low-fat mayonnaise

¼ cup low-fat buttermilk

2 tablespoons mustard

2 tablespoons lemon juice

1 tablespoon chopped fresh tarragon leaves

2 large Granny Smith apples, chopped

3 cups shredded red cabbage

3 cups shredded green cabbage

½ cup walnut pieces, toasted

Walnuts

Walnut pieces are larger than chopped walnuts but smaller than whole. To toast walnuts, spread them evenly on a cookie sheet and bake at 350°F for 10–15 minutes, shaking pan once or twice during baking time, until nuts are fragrant and turn a deeper golden-brown color. Cool completely before using.

1. In a large bowl, combine the yogurt, mayonnaise, buttermilk, mustard, lemon juice, and tarragon leaves and mix well to blend.

2. Add chopped apples, red cabbage, and green cabbage and mix well.

3. Cover, and chill in refrigerator for 2–4 hours before serving. Sprinkle with walnuts before serving.

PER SERVING: Calories: 136 | Protein: 4 g | Carbohydrates: 27 g | Fat: 6.9 g | Saturated Fat: 0.8 g | Cholesterol: 3 mg | Sodium: 133 mg | Potassium: 325 mg | Phosphorus: 109 mg | Calcium: 114 mg | Fiber: 3 g | Exchanges: ½ Fruit, 1½ Vegetable, 1½ Fat | Gluten Free: Use gluten-free mayonnaise and mustard

"Eggless" Salad Sandwich Spread

Tofu's mild flavor can be seasoned many ways.
Use different spices and cheeses to vary this spread recipe.

Tofu

The best tofu to use for fake egg-salad sandwich spread is firm or extra firm, depending on the consistency you like. Be sure to drain it very well; in fact, you can let it stand in a strainer for 30–40 minutes before using. If you don't, the excess liquid in the tofu will ruin the sandwich spread.

1. Drain the tofu, then drain again on paper towels, pressing to remove moisture. Set aside.

2. In a medium bowl, combine remaining ingredients and stir gently to combine.

3. Crumble the tofu into the bowl and mix until the mixture looks like egg salad.

4. Cover tightly, and refrigerate for 2–3 hours before serving. Store, covered, in the refrigerator for 3–4 days.

PER SERVING: Calories: 149 | Protein: 11 g | Carbohydrates: 5 g | Fat: 10.1 g | Saturated Fat: 2.0 g | Cholesterol: 9 mg | Sodium: 246 mg | Potassium: 209 mg | Phosphorus: 125 mg | Calcium: 161 mg | Fiber: 1 g | Exchanges: 1 Vegetable, 1 Lean Meat, 1½ Fat | Gluten Free: Use gluten-free mayonnaise, tofu, and mustard

Warm Broccoli and Potato Salad

This filling salad makes a delicious lunch for a winter afternoon.

INGREDIENTS | SERVES 8

6 medium-sized potatoes, peeled and cubed

2 cups broccoli florets

¼ cup fresh orange juice

3 tablespoons white wine or champagne vinegar

½ teaspoon dried basil

1 clove garlic, minced

⅛ teaspoon dried red pepper flakes

2 teaspoons dried parsley

⅛ teaspoon mustard powder

¼ teaspoon Dijon mustard

3 tablespoons extra-virgin olive oil

3 medium green onions, white and green parts thinly sliced

1. Preheat oven to lowest temperature.

2. Place the potatoes in a saucepan and cover with cold water. Bring to a boil, cover, and cook for 10 minutes, or until fork tender. Remove the potatoes with a slotted spoon. Save the water, keeping the pan on the heat. Transfer the potatoes to a baking sheet and place in the warm oven.

3. Add the broccoli to the reserved water and blanch for 1 minute. Remove the broccoli with a slotted spoon and add to the potatoes in the oven.

4. In a small saucepan over medium-high heat, combine the orange juice, vinegar, basil, garlic, and dried red pepper flakes and bring to a boil. Remove from the heat and whisk in the parsley, mustard powder, mustard, and olive oil. Add the onions and stir to mix.

5. Remove the vegetables from the oven and transfer to a serving bowl. Toss with the dressing, making sure all the potatoes and broccoli florets are thoroughly coated. Serve immediately.

PER SERVING: Calories: 181 | Protein: 4 g | Carbohydrates: 31 g | Fat: 5.3 g | Saturated Fat: 0.8 g | Cholesterol: 0 mg | Sodium: 17 mg | Potassium: 783 mg | Phosphorus: 110 mg | Calcium: 43 mg | Fiber: 4 g | Exchanges: 1½ Starch, 1 Vegetable, 1 Fat | Gluten Free: Use gluten-free mustard

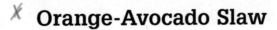

Orange-Avocado Slaw

This healthy and nutritious salad is a crowd-pleaser.
Try it at your next summer cookout instead of the traditional cole claw.

INGREDIENTS | SERVES 10

¼ cup fresh orange juice
½ teaspoon curry powder
⅛ teaspoon ground cumin
¼ teaspoon sugar
1 teaspoon white wine vinegar
1 tablespoon olive oil
4 cups grated broccoli
1 cup grated carrots
1 avocado, peeled and chopped
¼ teaspoon sea salt
Freshly ground black pepper, to taste

1. In a bowl, whisk together the orange juice, curry powder, cumin, sugar, and vinegar.

2. Add the oil in a stream, whisking until emulsified.

3. In a large bowl, toss the broccoli, carrots, and avocado. Drizzle with the vinaigrette.

4. Chill until ready to serve, and season with salt and pepper, if desired.

PER SERVING: Calories: 66 | Protein: 2 g | Carbohydrates: 6 g | Fat: 4.6 g | Saturated Fat: 0.7 g | Cholesterol: 0 mg | Sodium: 80 mg | Potassium: 267 mg | Phosphorus: 41 mg | Calcium: 27 mg | Fiber: 3 g | Exchanges: 1 Vegetable, 1 Fat | Gluten Free

Is There Any Fat in Fruit?

There is no fat in most varieties of fruit. Two exceptions are avocado and coconut. The fat contained in avocado is a combination of monounsaturated and polyunsaturated fats, which are considered healthy fats.

Cashew-Garlic Ranch Dressing

The combination of cashews and garlic is wonderful and makes a delicious addition to any salad.

INGREDIENTS | 8 SERVINGS

⅛ cup unsalted cashew butter

½ cup water

½ teaspoon stone-ground mustard

1½ tablespoons chili sauce

½ teaspoon horseradish

1 teaspoon tamari sauce

1 clove garlic

1½ teaspoons honey

⅛ teaspoon pepper

1. Process the cashew butter and water together in a blender or food processor until creamy.

2. Add the remaining ingredients and mix well. Refrigerate for 30 minutes.

PER SERVING: (⅛ of recipe): | Calories: 56 | Protein: 2 g | Carbohydrates: 4 g | Fat: 4 g | Saturated Fat: 0.8 g | Cholesterol: 0 mg | Sodium: 49 mg | Potassium: 61 mg | Phosphorus: 40 mg | Calcium: 6 mg | Fiber: 0 g | Exchanges: ½ Vegetable, 1 Fat | Gluten Free: Use gluten-free mustard, chili sauce, and tamari sauce

CHAPTER 16

Salsas, Sauces, and Condiments

Salsa with a Kick

The Tabasco sauce and cayenne pepper add kick.
You may add more if desired!

INGREDIENTS | 10 SERVINGS; SERVING SIZE APPROXIMATELY 2 OUNCES

2 teaspoons ground flaxseed

4 medium tomatoes, chopped

1 clove garlic, chopped

¼ cup chopped onion

½ tablespoon cider vinegar

¼ teaspoon Tabasco sauce

⅛ teaspoon ground cayenne pepper

1 tablespoon chopped fresh coriander

Place all the ingredients in a blender or food processor and process briefly, until blended but not smooth.

PER SERVING: (1/10 of recipe): | Calories: 14 | Protein: 1 g | Carbohydrates: 3 g | Fat: 0.3 g | Saturated Fat: 0 g | Cholesterol: 0 mg | Sodium: 4 mg | Potassium: 129 mg | Phosphorus: 17 mg | Calcium: 8 mg | Fiber: 1 g | Exchanges: ½ Vegetable | Gluten Free

Orange Sesame Dressing

Serve this flavorful, citrusy dressing over fish, vegetables, or rice.

INGREDIENTS | SERVES 2

1 tablespoon black or tan sesame seeds, toasted

1 tablespoon lemon juice

1 tablespoon sesame oil

2 teaspoons low-sodium soy sauce

2 tablespoons orange juice

1 clove roasted garlic, minced

Pinch of ginger (optional)

1. Grind sesame seeds in a suribachi bowl or food processor to make a paste.

2. Add remaining ingredients and mix together.

PER SERVING: Calories: 49 | Protein: 1 g | Carbohydrates: 5 g | Fat: 2.2 g | Saturated Fat: 0.3 g | Cholesterol: 0 mg | Sodium: 181 mg | Potassium: 68 mg | Phosphorus: 46 mg | Calcium: 12 mg | Fiber: 1 g | Exchanges: 1 Fat | Gluten Free: Use gluten-free soy sauce

High-Fiber Guacamole

Lima beans and peas add fiber to this delicious low-fat guacamole.
Remember that avocados have lots of heart-healthy monounsaturated fat and are low in saturated fat.

INGREDIENTS | SERVES 12

1 tablespoon olive oil

1 small onion, finely chopped

3 cloves garlic, minced

1 (10-ounce) package frozen baby lima beans

1 cup frozen peas

2 Florida avocados

2 tablespoons lemon juice

¼ teaspoon salt

½ cup low-fat sour cream

½ teaspoon crushed red pepper flakes

Keeping Guacamole Green

Guacamole turns brown because compounds in its cells oxidize when exposed to air. This is called enzymatic browning. To prevent this, you can either add an acidic ingredient like lemon juice to slow down the enzymes or limit air exposure. When covering guacamole, press plastic wrap directly on its surface to limit exposure to air.

1. In a medium saucepan, heat the olive oil over medium heat. Add the onion and garlic and cook and stir until crisp-tender, about 4 minutes.

2. Add the lima beans and cook and stir for 3 minutes, then add peas. Cook and stir for 2–4 minutes longer, until the peas and lima beans are hot and tender. Remove from heat and let cool for 20 minutes.

3. Peel the avocado, cut it in half, remove the pit, place it in a medium bowl, and top with lemon juice and salt.

4. Add the lima bean mixture to the avocado and mash with a potato masher or fork.

5. Blend in the sour cream and red pepper flakes. Serve immediately, or cover and refrigerate up to 4 hours before serving.

PER SERVING: Calories: 160 | Protein: 4 g | Carbohydrates: 13 g | Fat: 11.2 g | Saturated Fat: 2.8 g | Cholesterol: 10 mg | Sodium: 91 mg | Potassium: 435 mg | Phosphorus: 79 mg | Calcium: 51 mg | Fiber: 5 g | Exchanges: 1 Starch, 2 Fat | Gluten Free: Use gluten-free lima beans

Apple Butter

Granny Smith is the apple of choice for this recipe because of its tartness and texture. However, you can use other varieties, such as Macintosh or a mixture. The concentrated apple pulp adds rich fiber and flavor to your morning muffin or toast.

INGREDIENTS | SERVES 16

8 cups unpeeled apples, cored and sliced

1⅓ cups apple cider

1 cup brown sugar, unpacked

⅛ teaspoon salt

2 teaspoons cinnamon

¼ teaspoon ground cloves

½ teaspoon allspice

¼ cup brandy

Granny Smith

One of the world's most famous apple varieties, Granny Smiths are bright green and shiny. They are very juicy, and have a slightly tangy flavor. Granny Smiths were first cultivated in Australia in 1865 by Marie Ana Smith. They slowly made their way around the world, reaching the United States more than 100 years after they were first cultivated.

1. Combine the apples and apple cider in a large pot. Cover and cook over medium heat for 20 minutes, stirring frequently.

2. Purée the apples and liquid in a food mill and return to the pot.

3. Add the brown sugar, salt, cinnamon, cloves, and allspice to the apple purée and cook uncovered over low heat for 3 hours. Stir often, especially toward the end of the cooking time, to prevent sticking and burning.

4. Stir in brandy and remove from heat.

5. Ladle or pour the apple butter into hot sterilized jars, filling to ¼" from the top. Wipe jar rims. Cover at once with metal lids and screw-on bands. Let cool at room temperature, and refrigerate.

PER SERVING: Calories: 60 | Protein: 0 g | Carbohydrates: 13 g | Fat: 0.1 g | Saturated Fat: 0 g | Cholesterol: 0 mg | Sodium: 15 mg | Potassium: 65 mg | Phosphorus: 6 mg | Calcium: 9 mg | Fiber: 1 g | Exchanges: 1 Fruit | Gluten Free

Mango Chutney

Sweet and spicy, somewhere between preserves, pickles, and hot sauce, mango chutney complements Indian food perfectly. It's also a nice high-fiber dip for cold shrimp cocktail.

INGREDIENTS | SERVES 14

¾ cup sugar

¾ cup white wine vinegar

2 medium mangoes

1 garlic clove, peeled

¼ small green pepper

½ small onion

2 tablespoons grated fresh ginger

½ teaspoon white pepper

¼ teaspoon ground cinnamon

⅛ teaspoon ground cumin

Pinch of ground cloves

1. Combine the sugar and vinegar in a nonreactive saucepan and heat over low until sugar dissolves, about 5–10 minutes.

2. Peel and dice the mangoes, mince the garlic, and chop the green pepper and onion.

3. Add them to the pan along with the ginger, white pepper, cinnamon, cumin, and cloves.

4. Turn the heat up and simmer for 30 minutes, stirring occasionally.

5. Remove from heat, and refrigerate in a covered container.

PER SERVING: Calories: 64 | Protein: 0 g | Carbohydrates: 16 g | Fat: 0 g | Saturated Fat: 0 g | Cholesterol: 0 mg | Sodium: 6 mg | Potassium: 103 mg | Phosphorus: 9 mg | Calcium: 15 mg | Fiber: 1 g | Exchanges: 1 Fruit | Gluten Free

Chutneys

The flavor options for chutney are endless. The English brought the concept of a sweet and sour, spicy and hot, savory and highly textured fruit mixture back to Europe from India during the Raj. Nuts and onions can also be added to chutney. Mangoes are a favorite East Indian ingredient. Mixing fresh and dried fruits give the chutney great texture, extra sweetness, and fiber.

Multipurpose Garlic Spread

*Substituting other kinds of mustard will change the taste.
Don't be afraid to experiment with your favorite kind!*

INGREDIENTS | SERVES 8

1 ounce grated Parmesan cheese
4 cloves roasted garlic
1 teaspoon Dijon mustard
1 teaspoon dry white wine
½ teaspoon Worcestershire sauce
Pinch freshly ground black pepper
½ cup silken firm tofu
1 tablespoon extra-virgin olive oil

1. Put the grated cheese in a blender.

2. Add the garlic, mustard, wine, Worcestershire sauce, pepper, and tofu and blend until smooth.

3. While the blender is running, drizzle in the olive oil and continue to process until mixed with the other ingredients.

PER SERVING: Calories: 43 | Protein: 3 g | Carbohydrates: 1 g | Fat: 3.1 g | Saturated Fat: 0.9 g | Cholesterol: 3 mg | Sodium: 72 mg | Potassium: 42 mg | Phosphorus: 42 mg | Calcium:48 mg | Fiber: 0 g | Exchanges: ½ Lean Meat, ½ Fat | Gluten Free: Use gluten-free Worcestershire sauce, mustard, and tofu

Berry Good Salsa

This is a delicious salsa that uses summer fruits.
Try it for your next summer party!

INGREDIENTS | SERVES 16

1 cup fresh blackberries

½ medium cantaloupe, diced

1 jalapeño or banana pepper, diced

1 small red or green bell pepper, diced

1 medium-size red onion, diced

1 tablespoon lemon juice

⅛ teaspoon freshly ground black pepper

Pinch mustard powder

½ teaspoon lemon juice

½ teaspoon dried cilantro or parsley

½ teaspoon chili powder

Place all the ingredients in a food processor and process until well mixed. Do not overprocess—the salsa should remain somewhat chunky.

PER SERVING: Calories: 23 | Protein: 1 g | Carbohydrates: 6 g | Total fat: 0.2 g | Saturated Fat: 0 g | Cholesterol: 0 mg | Sodium: 13 mg | Potassium: 132 mg | Phosphorus: 13 mg | Calcium: 14 mg | Fiber: 1 g | Exchanges: ½ Fruit | Gluten Free

Mock Sour Cream

Nonfat yogurt and cottage cheese give a delicious flavor without the guilt!

INGREDIENTS	SERVES 6

⅛ cup plain nonfat yogurt
¼ cup 1%-fat cottage cheese
½ teaspoon vinegar

Vinegar Options

The type of vinegar used in the Mock Sour Cream recipe will affect the "tang" of the sour cream taste. Apple cider vinegar, for example, has a stronger taste; white wine or champagne vinegar tends to be milder.

Put all the ingredients in a blender or food processor and process until smooth.

PER SERVING: Calories: 10 | Protein: 1 g | Carbohydrate: 1 g | Fat: 0.1 g | Saturated Fat: 0.1 g | Cholesterol: 1 mg | Sodium: 42 mg | Potassium: 20 mg | Phosphorus: 20 mg | Calcium: 15 mg | Fiber: 0 g | Exchanges: 1 serving = Free Food | Gluten Free

X Chili Sauce

If your garden is overflowing with tomatoes, you can blanch, peel, and throw them into the recipe.

INGREDIENTS | SERVES 16

2 (28-ounce) cans low-sodium whole Italian plum tomatoes, drained

1 (6-ounce) can unsalted tomato paste

1 tablespoon garlic powder

1 tablespoon onion powder

1 tablespoon chili powder, or to taste

1 teaspoon ground cloves

½ teaspoon ground cinnamon

4 teaspoons no-calorie sweetener such as Splenda

4 unpacked teaspoons brown sugar

1 teaspoon salt

1 teaspoon freshly ground black pepper, or to taste

1. Mix all the ingredients in a large, heavy-bottomed pot. Bring to a boil, reduce heat, and simmer with the cover slightly cracked.

2. Stirring occasionally, simmer for about 3 hours, or until the sauce is reduced by one-half. Cool, jar for storage, and refrigerate.

PER SERVING: Calories: 30 | Protein: 1 g | Carbohydrates: 7 g | Fat: 0.3 g | Saturated Fat: 0.0 g | Cholesterol: 0 mg | Sodium: 169 mg | Potassium: 266 mg | Phosphorus: 28 mg | Calcium: 32 mg | Fiber: 2 g | Exchanges: 1 Vegetable | Gluten Free

Your Own Sauces

Once you have made a sauce base, you can taste and adjust the ingredients. Maybe you'd like more sour, spicy, salty, or sweet. Putting your own stamp on a recipe is the fun part of cooking. It puts you, the cook, in control!

Homemade Sugar-Free Chocolate Sauce

This sauce will keep nicely in the refrigerator.
Use it as a base for other desserts or spoon it over ice cream and frozen yogurt.

INGREDIENTS | SERVES 4

⅓ cup Dutch process cocoa

2 tablespoons no-calorie sweetener such as Splenda, or to taste

¼ teaspoon salt

1 tablespoon cornstarch

1 teaspoon instant espresso

1 cup cold water

1. Whisk all the ingredients together until all of the lumps are gone.

2. Place in a saucepan over medium heat. Bring to a boil, whisking until thickened, about 10–15 minutes. Taste and add more sweetener if necessary.

3. Let cool, and pour into a jar for use as needed.

PER SERVING: Calories: 27 | Protein: 1 g | Carbohydrates: 7 g | Fat: 1 g | Saturated Fat: 0.6 g | Cholesterol: 0 mg | Sodium: 149 mg | Potassium: 192 mg | Phosphorus: 54 mg | Calcium: 10 mg | Fiber: 2 g | Exchanges: ½ Fruit | Gluten Free: Use gluten-free espresso

Apple, Cranberry, and Walnut Chutney

This is excellent with duckling, chicken, and, of course, turkey.
It's easy to make, and can be frozen.

INGREDIENTS | SERVES 16

½ cup finely chopped shallots

2 tablespoons canola oil

2 cups cranberries, fresh or frozen, washed and picked over if fresh

2 tart medium apples, peeled, cored, and chopped

½ unpacked cup brown sugar, or to taste

¼ cup cider vinegar

2 ounces water

1 teaspoon orange zest

½ teaspoon ground coriander seed

½ teaspoon black pepper

½ teaspoon salt

½ cup walnut pieces, toasted

1. In a large, heavy saucepan, cook the shallots in oil until softened.

2. Mix everything but the walnuts in with the shallots. Cook, stirring, until berries have popped and the sauce has become very thick, about 10–15 minutes.

3. Cool, and stir in toasted walnut pieces. Store in the refrigerator, or freeze.

PER SERVING: Calories: 74 | Protein: 1 g | Carbohydrates: 10 g | Fat: 3.9 g | Saturated Fat: 0.3 g | Cholesterol: 0 mg | Sodium: 75 mg | Potassium: 70 mg | Phosphorus: 19 mg | Calcium: 12 mg | Fiber: 1 g | Exchanges: ½ Fruit, 1 Fat | Gluten Free

Fruit and Pepper

Try putting some pepper on watermelon, cantaloupe, or honeydew melon. You'll find that peppery chutneys and salsas make an excellent accompaniment to all kinds of dishes.

Hollandaise-Style Sauce

This sauce is an excellent addition to Eggs Benedict.

INGREDIENTS | SERVES 10

½ cup light mayonnaise

1 tablespoon fresh lemon juice

2 tablespoons reduced-calorie honey mustard dressing

⅛ teaspoon dried red pepper flakes, crushed

Freshly ground black pepper, to taste

1. Add all the ingredients to a small serving bowl and whisk to combine.

2. Refrigerate leftovers. This sauce can be safely kept, covered, in the refrigerator for several days.

PER SERVING: Calories: 46 | Protein: 0 g | Carbohydrates: 2 g | Fat: 4.3 g | Saturated Fat: 0.7 g | Cholesterol: 4 mg | Sodium: 108 mg | Potassium: 12 mg | Phosphorus: 6 mg | Calcium: 3 mg | Fiber: 0 g | Exchanges: 1 Fat | Gluten Free: Use gluten-free mayonnaise and salad dressing

CHAPTER 17

Breads and Muffins

Whole-Wheat Zucchini Bread

Add dry fruits or nuts to this bread to add sweetness, crunch, and depth of flavor.

INGREDIENTS | SERVES 20

2 large eggs

2 ounces egg whites

½ cup honey

2 cups zucchini, shredded

⅔ cup unsweetened applesauce

⅓ cup canola oil

2 teaspoons vanilla

2 cups whole-wheat pastry flour

1 cup all-purpose flour

¼ cup no-calorie granular sweetener such as Splenda Granular

1 teaspoon salt

2 teaspoons low-sodium baking powder

1 teaspoon baking soda

2 teaspoons cinnamon

½ teaspoons nutmeg

⅓ cup hulled unsalted sunflower seeds, toasted

Variations

For variation on this recipe, ⅓ cup dried cranberries, currants, raisins, or chopped nuts can be added in place of the sunflower seeds.

1. Preheat oven to 350°F. Spray 4 aluminum mini loaf pans with cooking spray.

2. In a large mixing bowl, beat the egg and egg whites until foamy. Mix in the honey, zucchini, applesauce, canola oil, and vanilla.

3. In a separate mixing bowl, sift together the whole-wheat flour, all-purpose flour, sweetener, salt, baking powder, baking soda, cinnamon, and nutmeg.

4. Gradually add the dry ingredients to the zucchini mixture and mix until all ingredients are combined, but do not overmix. Stir in sunflower seeds.

5. Divide the batter evenly into prepared mini loaf pans. Bake for 35–40 minutes, or until tops are browned and an inserted toothpick comes out clean.

6. Remove pans to a wire rack and cool for 10 minutes before removing from pans. Cool completely before slicing.

PER SERVING: Calories: 154 | Protein: 3 g | Carbohydrates: 25 g | Fat: 4.9 g | Saturated Fat: 0.4 g | Cholesterol: 0 mg | Sodium: 192 mg | Potassium: 141 mg | Phosphorus: 83 mg | Calcium: 32 mg | Fiber: 1 g | Exchanges: 1½ Starch, ½ Fat | Gluten Free: This recipe cannot be made gluten free

Banana-Blueberry Oatmeal Bread

Quick breads are easy to make. Their flavor and texture usually gets better if allowed to stand, covered, overnight at room temperature.

INGREDIENTS | SERVES 12

1 (3-ounce) package low-fat cream cheese, softened
¼ unpacked cup brown sugar
¼ cup sugar
2 medium bananas, mashed
1 large egg
2 egg whites from large eggs
¼ cup orange juice
1 cup all-purpose flour
½ cup whole-wheat flour
1 teaspoon baking powder
1 teaspoon baking soda
1 cup blueberries
½ cup regular oatmeal

1. Preheat oven to 350°F. Spray a 9" × 5" loaf pan with nonstick cooking spray containing flour, and set aside.

2. In a large bowl, combine the cream cheese with the brown sugar and sugar and beat until fluffy. Beat in the mashed bananas, then add the egg, egg whites, and orange juice and beat until smooth.

3. Stir together the flour, whole-wheat flour, baking powder, and baking soda. Add to the batter and stir just until combined. Fold in the blueberries and oatmeal. Pour into prepared loaf pan.

4. Bake for 50–60 minutes, or until the bread is a deep golden brown and a toothpick inserted in the center comes out clean. Remove from pan and cool on wire rack.

PER SERVING: Calories: 144 | Protein: 4 g | Carbohydrates: 29 g | Fat: 1.9 g | Saturated Fat: 0.9 g | Cholesterol: 22 mg | Sodium: 196 mg | Potassium: 172 mg | Phosphorus: 75 mg | Calcium: 45 mg | Fiber: 2 g | Exchanges: 1½ Starch, ½ Fruit | Gluten Free: Use gluten-free flour, oatmeal, baking powder, and cream cheese

Fresh or Frozen Fruit?

When baking, you can usually use either fresh or frozen fruit. If using frozen fruit, do not thaw before adding it to the batter, or it will add too much liquid and color or stain the bread. Use frozen fruits that are dry packed, with no added sugar or other ingredients.

Savory Herb Muffins

These little muffins are delicious served with soup for lunch on a cold day.

1 cup nonfat buttermilk

1 large egg

2 large egg whites

5 tablespoons canola oil

2 tablespoons chopped fresh rosemary leaves

2 teaspoons fresh thyme leaves

2 tablespoons chopped flat-leaf parsley

¼ teaspoon dried marjoram

¼ cup grated Parmesan cheese

½ cup cornmeal

1¼ cups all-purpose flour

½ cup whole-wheat flour

1 teaspoon baking powder

1 teaspoon baking soda

Rosemary

Rosemary is one of the herbs believed to reduce arterial inflammation. Try to find fresh rosemary; dried rosemary is so stiff and brittle it has to be chopped very finely or it can be difficult to swallow. To use fresh rosemary, pull the thin leaves backward from the stem, then pile up and chop with a chef's knife.

1. Preheat oven to 375°F. Place paper liners into 12 muffin cups and set aside.

2. In a large bowl, combine the buttermilk, egg, egg whites, canola oil, all the herbs, Parmesan, and cornmeal and mix well until combined. Add the flour, whole-wheat flour, baking powder, and baking soda and stir just until dry ingredients are moistened.

3. Fill prepared muffin cups ⅔ full. Bake for 20–25 minutes, or until muffins are light golden brown and set. Remove from muffin cups, and serve warm.

PER SERVING: Calories: 161 | Protein: 5 g | Carbohydrates: 19 g | Fat: 7.5 g | Saturated Fat: 1.1 g | Cholesterol: 20 mg | Sodium: 217 mg | Potassium: 103 mg | Phosphorus: 95 mg | Calcium: 79 mg | Fiber: 1 g | Exchanges: 1½ Starch, 1 Fat | Gluten Free: Use gluten-free flour, cornmeal, and baking powder

Cranberry Cornmeal Muffins

Masa harina is corn flour; it's not the same as cornmeal.
You can find it in the international foods aisle of the supermarket.

INGREDIENTS | SERVES 12

½ cup cornmeal

½ cup masa harina

1 cup all-purpose flour

2 tablespoons crushed flaxseed

¼ unpacked cup brown sugar

1 teaspoon baking powder

1 teaspoon baking soda

1 large egg

¼ cup canola oil

1 cup nonfat buttermilk

1 teaspoon grated orange zest

2 tablespoons honey

1 teaspoon vanilla extract

⅓ cup chopped cranberries

⅓ cup dried cranberries

1. Preheat oven to 400°F. Line 12 muffin cups with paper liners and set aside.

2. In a large bowl, combine the cornmeal, masa harina, flour, flaxseed, brown sugar, baking powder, and baking soda and mix well.

3. In a small bowl, combine the egg, oil, buttermilk, orange zest, honey, and vanilla and beat to combine. Add to the dry ingredients and stir just until moistened. Add chopped and dried cranberries.

4. Fill muffin cups ⅔ full. Bake for 15–22 minutes, or until toothpick inserted in center comes out clean. Let cool on wire racks for 10 minutes before serving.

PER SERVING: Calories: 168 | Protein: 3 g | Carbohydrates: 26 g | Fat: 6.1 g | Saturated Fat: 0.7 g | Cholesterol: 18 mg | Sodium: 177 mg | Potassium: 96 mg | Phosphorus: 77 mg | Calcium: 64 mg | Fiber: 2 g | Exchanges: 1 Starch, ¾ Fruit, 1 Fat | Gluten Free: Use gluten-free baking powder and flour

Oat Bran Dinner Rolls

These excellent rolls are light yet hearty, with a wonderful flavor and a bit of crunch.

INGREDIENTS | SERVES 30

1½ cups water

¾ cup quick-cooking oats

½ cup oat bran

¼ unpacked cup brown sugar

2 tablespoons plant sterol margarine

1 cup buttermilk

2 (¼-ounce) packages active dry yeast

2½ cups all-purpose flour, divided

1½ cups whole-wheat flour

½ teaspoon salt

2 tablespoons honey

1 large egg white, beaten

2 tablespoons oat bran

1. In a medium saucepan, bring water to a boil over high heat. Add the oats, oat bran, brown sugar, and margarine and stir until margarine melts. Remove from heat and let cool to lukewarm.

2. Meanwhile, in a microwave-safe glass cup, microwave the buttermilk on medium for 1 minute, or until lukewarm (about 110°F). Sprinkle the yeast over the milk, stir, and let stand for 10 minutes.

3. In a large mixing bowl, combine 1 cup all-purpose flour, whole-wheat flour, and salt. Add the honey, cooled oatmeal mixture, and softened yeast mixture and beat until smooth. Gradually add enough remaining all-purpose flour to form a soft dough.

4. Turn onto a lightly floured board and knead until smooth and elastic, about 5–7 minutes. Place in a greased bowl, turning to grease the top. Cover and let rise for 1 hour, or until dough doubles.

5. Punch down the dough and divide it into thirds. Divide each third into 10 pieces. Roll balls between your hands to smooth. Place balls into two 9" round cake pans. Brush with egg white and sprinkle with 2 tablespoons oat bran. Cover and let rise until doubled, about 45 minutes.

6. Preheat oven to 375°F. Bake rolls for 15–25 minutes, or until firm to the touch and golden brown. Remove from pans and cool on wire racks.

PER SERVING: Calories: 88 | Protein: 3 g | Carbohydrates: 18 g | Fat: 1.0 g | Saturated Fat: 0.2 g | Cholesterol: 0 mg | Sodium: 57 mg | Potassium: 81 mg | Phosphorus: 70 mg | Calcium: 17 mg | Fiber: 2 g | Exchanges: 1 Starch | Gluten Free: This recipe cannot be made gluten free

Three-Grain French Bread

Yogurt and orange juice add a bit of sourdough texture and flavor to this easy and delicious loaf.

INGREDIENTS | SERVES 16

¾ cup warm water

2 (¼-ounce) packages active dry yeast

1 tablespoon sugar

¼ cup orange juice

1 cup plain yogurt

2 tablespoons lemon juice

1 large egg

⅓ cup oat bran

½ teaspoon salt

1½ cups whole-wheat flour

3¼ cups bread flour

1 tablespoon cornmeal

Storing French Bread

Homemade French bread will not last very long after it's baked. Within two days of baking the bread, slice into 1" slices and flash freeze on a cookie sheet. When bread is frozen, pack into hard-sided containers, label, seal, and freeze up to 3 months. To use, spread with olive oil and toast right out of the freezer.

1. In a large bowl, combine the water, yeast, and sugar. Stir and let stand for 10 minutes. Add the orange juice, yogurt, lemon juice, and egg and beat for 1 minute. Add the oat bran, salt, whole-wheat flour, and 1 cup bread flour and beat. Cover for 1 hour.

2. Gradually add enough remaining bread flour to form a firm dough. Turn onto a floured surface and knead for 10 minutes, until smooth and elastic. Place in a greased bowl, turning to grease the top. Cover and let rise for 1 hour.

3. Punch down the dough and let it rest for 10 minutes. With nonstick cooking spray, spray two 14" × 4" rectangles on a cookie sheet and sprinkle with cornmeal. Divide the dough in half and roll each half to a 14" × 6" rectangle. Roll up tightly, starting at longer side. Pinch edges and ends to seal and place, seam-side down, on the prepared cookie sheet.

4. Cover and let rise for 30 minutes, or until doubled.

5. Preheat oven to 375°F. Slash the bread in shallow cuts several times, cutting across the loaves, using a sharp knife. Bake for 30–40 minutes, or until the loaves are golden brown and sound hollow when tapped with your fingers. Let cool on wire rack.

PER SERVING: Calories: 158 | Protein: 6 g | Carbohydrates: 32 g | Fat: 1.1 g | Saturated Fat: 0.3 g | Cholesterol: 17 mg | Sodium: 414 mg | Potassium: 163 mg | Phosphorus: 250 mg | Calcium: 125 mg | Fiber: 3 g | Exchanges: 2 Starch | Gluten Free: This recipe cannot be made gluten free

Raisin Bran Muffins

A breakfast of a glass of orange juice (with pulp!) and a bran muffin is a delicious way to start your day with fiber. The raisins add sweetness and fiber, and you can substitute whole-wheat flour for all-purpose flour to add even more fiber.

INGREDIENTS | SERVES 36

1 cup boiling water
2½ cups All-Bran cereal
2½ cups all-purpose flour
2½ teaspoons baking soda
1 teaspoon salt
½ cup canola oil
1 cup sugar
2 large eggs, beaten
2 cups nonfat buttermilk
1½ packed cups seedless raisins
1 cup bran flakes

1. Preheat oven to 400°F. Grease a muffin tin or line it with fluted paper cups. Pour the boiling water over 1 cup of All-Bran and let it sit for 10 minutes.

2. Mix the flour, baking soda, and salt in a mixing bowl and set aside.

3. Mix the oil into the All-Bran and water mixture, then add the remaining All-Bran, sugar, eggs, and buttermilk.

4. Add the flour mixture to the All-Bran mixture and mix to combine. Stir in the raisins and bran flakes.

5. Fill the muffin cups ¾ full with the batter and bake for 20 minutes.

PER SERVING: Calories: 125 | Protein: 3 g | Carbohydrates: 23 g | Fat: 3.8 g | Saturated Fat: 0.4 g | Cholesterol: 12 mg | Sodium: 194 mg | Potassium: 136 mg | Phosphorus: 92 mg | Calcium: 40 mg | Fiber: 2 g | Exchanges: 1 Starch, ½ Fruit, ½ Fat | Gluten Free: This recipe cannot be made gluten free

Quick Breads Versus Muffins

Most quick-bread recipes can be used for muffins. You will get 12 standard muffins or 24 mini muffins. Always prepare your muffin tins with nonstick spray, even those that are supposedly nonstick. Muffins bake in about 15–20 minutes, and make nice equal portions. Never overfill the muffin cups or they will rise and spill over the top.

Butternut Squash Cheese Muffins

This is a great way to get a serving of vegetables into your day.

INGREDIENTS | SERVES 12

1 tablespoon unsalted margarine (80% fat)

1 tablespoon extra-light olive oil or canola oil

1 cup chopped sweet onion

1 cup sliced button mushrooms

¼ cup water

2 cups cubed roasted butternut squash

6 tablespoons unbleached all-purpose flour

3 tablespoons wheat germ

2 large eggs

¼ teaspoon freshly ground black pepper

½ cup grated Jarlsberg cheese

1 tablespoon hulled sesame seeds

Roasting Butternut Squash

Preheat oven to 350°F. Wash the outside skin of the squash. Place the whole squash on a jelly roll pan or baking sheet. Pierce the skin a few times with a knife. Bake for 1 hour, or until tender. Once the squash is cool enough to handle, slice it open, scrape out the seeds, and scrape the squash pulp off of the skin.

1. Preheat oven to 400°F.

2. Add the margarine and oil to a nonstick sauté pan over high heat. When the mix begins to sizzle, reduce heat to medium and add the onion and mushrooms. Sauté until the onion is transparent, about 5–10 minutes. Set aside to cool.

3. In the bowl of a food processor or in a blender, combine the cooled sautéed mixture and all of the remaining ingredients except the cheese and sesame seeds and pulse until mixed.

4. Fold the cheese into the squash mixture. Spoon the resulting batter into muffin cups treated with nonstick spray or lined with foil muffin liners, filling each muffin section to the top. Evenly divide the sesame seeds over the top of the batter.

5. Bake for 35 to 40 minutes. For savory appetizers, make 24 mini-muffins and bake for 20 to 25 minutes.

PER SERVING: Calories: 80 | Protein: 4 g | Carbohydrates: 6 g | Fat: 4.8 g | Saturated Fat: 1.5 g | Cholesterol: 39 mg | Sodium: 28 mg | Potassium: 170 mg | Phosphorus: 89 mg | Calcium: 68 mg | Fiber: 1 g | Exchanges: 1 Vegetable, ½ Lean Meat, ½ Fat | Gluten Free: Replace wheat germ with gluten-free oat bran and use gluten-free flour and margarine

Lemon Pear Scones

These scones are the perfect way to help start a weekend morning!

INGREDIENTS | SERVES 12

1 cup dry oatmeal

1 cup unbleached all-purpose flour

⅓ cup plus 2 tablespoons granulated sugar

1½ teaspoons low-salt baking powder

½ teaspoon baking soda

1 teaspoon dried ground ginger

¼ teaspoon cinnamon

¼ teaspoon nutmeg

Pinch salt

2 teaspoons lemon zest

3 tablespoons unsalted tub margarine (80% fat)

⅔ cup plain nonfat yogurt

1 large egg, lightly beaten

1 teaspoon vanilla extract

2 teaspoons lemon extract

½ cup peeled and grated pear

Teatime Tip

You can underbake some of the scones and then, once they've cooled, wrap them in nonstick foil and freeze them until needed. When needed, pop the foil-wrapped scones into a preheated 350°F oven for 15–20 minutes.

1. Preheat oven to 400°. Treat a baking sheet or jelly roll pan with nonstick cooking spray.

2. In a large bowl, combine the oatmeal, flour, ⅓ cup of the sugar, baking powder, baking soda, ginger, cinnamon, nutmeg, salt, and lemon zest and mix well. Cut in the margarine until crumbly.

3. In a separate bowl, mix together the yogurt, beaten egg, vanilla extract, and lemon extract. Add to the dry ingredients, using a fork to mix the wet ingredients in to moisten the dry. Fold in the grated pear.

4. Drop ¼ cupfuls of batter in semiflattened mounds on the treated baking sheet. Sprinkle with the remaining sugar.

5. Bake for 16–18 minutes, until light golden brown. Serve warm.

PER SERVING: Calories: 135 | Protein: 3 g | Carbohydrates: 23 g | Fat: 3.6 g | Saturated Fat: 0.8 g | Cholesterol: 18 mg | Sodium: 83 mg | Potassium: 153 mg | Phosphorus: 108 mg | Calcium: 62 mg | Fiber: 1 g | Exchanges: 1 Starch, ½ Fruit, ½ Fat | Gluten Free: Use gluten-free oatmeal, flour, baking powder, margarine, and vanilla

Savory Summer Squash Bread

You can make several batches of this bread and freeze them to enjoy that fresh, summery taste any season.

INGREDIENTS | SERVES 12

2 large eggs

½ cup milk

1 cup zucchini or yellow summer squash, trimmed and grated

2 medium green onions, finely chopped

1 tablespoon melted unsalted margarine

1 teaspoon celery salt

½ teaspoon freshly ground black pepper

1 teaspoon no-calorie sweetener such as Splenda

¼ cup Italian flat-leaf parsley, minced

2 teaspoons chopped fresh summer savory or 1 teaspoon dried savory

1 teaspoon low-sodium baking powder

1 teaspoon baking soda

1 cup all-purpose flour

½ cup whole-wheat flour

1. Preheat oven to 350°F. Prepare a standard loaf pan with nonstick spray.

2. Whisk the eggs and milk together in a blender. Add the grated squash, green onions, and unsalted margarine and blend till combined.

3. Combine celery salt, pepper, sweetener, parsley, savory, baking powder, baking soda, and flours in a separate bowl. Add to moist ingredients and mix thoroughly.

4. Pour into the loaf pan and bake for 60 minutes. Remove the pan from the oven and cool loaf on a rack. This recipe is excellent with whipped cream cheese.

PER SERVING: Calories: 83 | Protein: 3 g | Carbohydrates: 13 g | Fat: 2.0 g | Saturated Fat: 0.5 g | Cholesterol: 35 mg | Sodium: 147 mg | Potassium: 142 mg | Phosphorus: 89 mg | Calcium: 49 mg | Fiber: 1 g | Exchanges: 1 Starch | Gluten Free: Use gluten-free flour, baking powder, and margarine

Herbs Make Food Savory

You can do a lot with herbs to make even the plainest dishes more appealing. For added zing, mix sweet and savory flavors. Most supermarkets carry a good selection of fresh herbs. You can also grow your own on a sunny windowsill or in your backyard and pick them as you need them.

Swedish Coffee Bread

This braided bread is a sweet Scandinavian delicacy.
It is particularly popular around the holiday season.

INGREDIENTS | SERVES 24

1 ounce live yeast, crumbled
½ cup warm skim milk
½ cup unsalted tub margarine
1 cup no-calorie sweetener such as Splenda, divided
1 teaspoon salt
3 large eggs, divided
½ cup cold milk
2 cups all-purpose flour
2 cups whole-wheat flour, plus extra for sprinkling
1 tablespoon ground cardamom
1 tablespoon ground cinnamon
1 cup packed seedless raisins
1 cup chopped walnuts

1. In a small bowl, mix the yeast and warm milk. Set aside.

2. In a large bowl, mix the margarine, ½ cup sweetener, and salt. Beat in 2 of the eggs and cold milk. Add the yeast, and set aside for 10 minutes.

3. Stir in the flours, mix well, cover, and let rise in a warm place for 60 minutes.

4. Sprinkle a flat surface with flour and roll the dough out onto it. Knead the dough until it is smooth and elastic. Roll into a long rope, about 18" long and ⅓" thick.

5. Mix ½ cup sweetener, cardamom, and cinnamon in a small bowl. Sprinkle the dough with the spice mixture, then spread the raisins and nuts on top. Spray a cookie sheet with nonstick spray.

6. Cut the dough in three 6" pieces. Braid the pieces together and place on the cookie sheet.

7. Cover and let rise for 60 minutes. When the dough has doubled in size, heat oven to 350°F. Beat the remaining egg. Brush the dough with egg and bake for 25–30 minutes.

PER SERVING: Calories: 179 | Protein: 5 g | Carbohydrates: 24 g | Fat: 8.0 g | Saturated Fat: 1.2 g | Cholesterol: 27 mg | Sodium: 114 mg | Potassium: 178 mg | Phosphorus: 108 mg | Calcium: 34 mg | Fiber: 3 g | Exchanges: 1 Starch, ½ Fruit, 1½ Fat | Gluten Free: Use gluten-free flour and margarine

Desserts

Carrot Fruit Cup

This is a lovely, colorful mixture of sweet carrots and fruit.

INGREDIENTS | SERVES 4

50 raisins
2 medium carrots, grated
1 medium apple, peeled and grated
1 tablespoon frozen apple juice concentrate
1 teaspoon cinnamon
Pinch of ginger
1 frozen banana (7½" long), sliced

1. Soak the raisins overnight in a little more than enough water to cover them.

2. When you're ready to prepare the dessert, drain the water from the raisins and pour them into a bowl.

3. Add the carrots and apple and stir in the frozen apple juice concentrate and spices until blended.

4. Add the banana slices and stir again. Chill until ready to serve.

PER SERVING: Calories: 82 | Protein: 1 g | Carbohydrates: 21 g | Fat: 0.3 g | Saturated Fat: 0.1 g | Cholesterol: 0 mg | Sodium: 23 mg | Potassium: 300 mg | Phosphorus: 29 mg | Calcium: 24 mg | Fiber: 3 g | Exchanges: 1½ Fruit | Gluten Free

Carrots for Dessert?

Carrots are naturally sweet. They will also add color to your dessert. Carrots are a great source of carotenoids, which turn into vitamin A in the body. In fact, carotenoids were named in honor of the carrot!

Lemon Mousse

Pear nectar is very mild, and it adds a nice bit of sweetness to this tart mousse.

INGREDIENTS | SERVES 4

1 (¼-ounce) envelope unflavored gelatin

¼ cup cold water

⅓ cup lemon juice

⅔ cup pear nectar

¼ cup sugar, divided

1 teaspoon grated lemon zest

1 cup nonfat lemon yogurt

2 ounces pasteurized egg whites

¼ teaspoon cream of tartar

Pasteurized Egg Whites

You can find pasteurized eggs in most grocery stores. Be sure to carefully abide by the sell-by and use-by dates that are stamped on the package and usually on each egg. Pasteurized egg whites take longer to whip to peaks than ordinary eggs. Just keep beating them until the peaks form. Cream of tartar helps stabilize the foam.

1. In a microwave-safe glass measuring cup, combine gelatin and cold water and let stand for 5 minutes to soften gelatin.

2. Stir in lemon juice, pear nectar, and 2 tablespoons sugar. Microwave on high for 1–2 minutes, stirring twice during cooking time, until sugar and gelatin completely dissolve. Stir in lemon zest, and let cool for 30 minutes.

3. When gelatin mixture is cool to the touch, blend in the lemon yogurt.

4. In a medium bowl, combine the egg whites with the cream of tartar and beat until soft peaks form. Gradually stir in the remaining 2 tablespoons of sugar, beating until stiff peaks form.

5. Fold the gelatin mixture into the egg whites until combined. Pour into serving glasses or goblets, cover, and chill until firm, about 4–6 hours.

PER SERVING: Calories: 147 | Protein: 6 g | Carbohydrates: 31 g | Fat: 0.2 g | Saturated Fat: 0.1 g | Cholesterol: 1 mg | Sodium: 74 mg | Potassium: 217 mg | Phosphorus: 91 mg | Calcium: 117 mg | Fiber: 0 g | Exchanges: 1¾ Fruit, ½ Skim Milk | Gluten Free: Use gluten-free pear nectar

Peach Melba Parfait

This fresh and easy dessert can be made with many flavor combinations.
Try sliced pears with orange yogurt and mandarin orange segments.

INGREDIENTS | SERVES 4

4 ripe medium peaches, peeled and sliced

1 tablespoon lemon juice

2 tablespoons sugar

1 cup nonfat raspberry yogurt

1 pint fresh raspberries

4 leaves fresh mint

Melba

Peach Melba is a dessert invented in the 1890s to honor the opera singer Nellie Melba. She loved ice cream but didn't like its effect on her vocal cords. The chef Escoffier created Peach Melba by combining peaches and raspberries into a warm syrup served over ice cream.

1. In a medium bowl, combine the peaches, lemon juice, and sugar and let stand for 10 minutes. Stir to dissolve sugar.

2. In 4 parfait or wine glasses, place some of the peach mixture. Top with a spoonful of the yogurt, then some fresh raspberries. Repeat layers, ending with raspberries.

3. Cover, and chill for 2–4 hours before serving. Garnish with mint sprig.

PER SERVING: Calories: 182 | Protein: 5 g | Carbohydrates: 42 g | Fat: 1.0 g | Saturated Fat: 0.1 g | Cholesterol: 1 mg | Sodium: 37 mg | Potassium: 526 mg | Phosphorus: 126 mg | Calcium: 122 mg | Fiber: 7 g | Exchanges: 2½ Fruit, ¼ Skim Milk | Gluten Free: Use gluten-free yogurt

Mango Sorbet

This tastes like fresh mangoes with a velvety texture. You can substitute lime juice for lemon for a different sparkle. Mangoes are high in fiber and vitamin A. Throw a few blueberries on top of each dish of sorbet for great color and even more fiber.

INGREDIENTS | SERVES 12

½ cup sugar

¼ cup water

3 cups mango purée

¼ cup lemon juice

Mango Purée

Choose very ripe mangos. Purée in a blender or a food processor, and add to recipes as needed.

1. Combine sugar and water in a saucepan and heat just until sugar dissolves. Remove from heat and chill.

2. Combine chilled sugar syrup, mango purée, and lemon juice.

3. Freeze in an ice-cream freezer according to manufacturer's instructions.

PER SERVING: Calories: 60 | Protein: 0 g | Carbohydrates: 16 g | Fat: 0.1 g | Saturated Fat: 0 g | Cholesterol: 0 mg | Sodium: 2 mg | Potassium: 70 mg | Phosphorus: 5 mg | Calcium: 5 mg | Fiber: 1 g | Exchanges: 1 Fruit | Gluten Free

Sesame Seed Cookies

These delicate cookies are a type of lace cookie, full of delicious and fiber-rich sesame seeds. The seeds also add a touch of protein. These cookies are elegant enough for dessert, topped with ice cream.

INGREDIENTS | SERVES 15

4½ teaspoons honey

1½ tablespoons tub margarine

½ cup sifted powdered sugar

1 tablespoon water

½ cup sesame seeds

Pinch of salt

2 tablespoons all-purpose flour

Learning about Seeds

Seeds are delicious, as well as high in both fiber and protein. However, people with diverticulitis or diverticulosis cannot eat them. Children and people without these diseases will benefit from a good daily dose of seeds in the diet. Eating nuts and seeds while you're healthy will help prevent intestinal problems.

1. Stir the honey, margarine, powdered sugar, and water together in a saucepan. Turn the heat to medium and bring to a boil. Boil for 1 minute, and remove from heat.

2. Stir in the sesame seeds, salt, and flour and let cool to room temperature.

3. Preheat oven to 350°F. Line baking sheets with parchment paper or silicone mats.

4. Roll the cookie dough into balls and place them 4" apart from each other on the prepared baking sheets.

5. Bake for 8 minutes, then let cool on racks. Peel off the cooled cookies and store in an airtight container.

PER SERVING: Calories: 62 | Protein: 1 g | Carbohydrates: 7 g | Fat: 3.6 g | Saturated Fat: 0.6 g | Cholesterol: 0 mg | Sodium: 22 mg | Potassium: 23 mg | Phosphorus: 40 mg | Calcium: 7 mg | Fiber: 1 | Exchanges: ½ Starch, ½ Fat | Gluten Free: Use gluten-free flour and margarine

Steamed Raspberry Lemon Custard

Garnish these individual desserts with raspberries, mint, and a dusting of powdered sugar, if desired.

INGREDIENTS | SERVES 4

2 large eggs

¼ teaspoon cream of tartar

Zest and juice of 1 lemon

¼ teaspoon pure lemon extract or vanilla extract

3 tablespoons unbleached all-purpose flour

¼ cup granulated sugar

40 fresh raspberries

Steaming Savvy

To steam custards at the same time with other dishes that might affect taste, wrap the ramekins in plastic wrap so they won't pick up the other aromas and put them in the top tier of the steamer.

1. Separate the egg yolks and whites. Add the egg whites to a large bowl and set aside the yolks.

2. Use an electric mixer or wire whisk to beat the egg whites until frothy. Add the cream of tartar and continue to whip or whisk until soft peaks form.

3. In a small bowl, mix together the lemon zest, lemon juice, lemon extract, flour, sugar, and egg yolks and gently fold into the whites with a spatula.

4. Treat 4 6-ounce ramekins with nonstick spray. Place 10 raspberries in the bottom of each. Spoon the batter into the ramekins and set them in a steamer with a lid. Cover and steam for 15–20 minutes.

5. To remove the custards from the ramekins, run a thin knife around the edges and turn upside down onto plates.

PER SERVING: Calories: 123 | Protein: 4 g | Carbohydrates: 23 g | Fat: 2.7 g | Saturated Fat: 0.8 g | Cholesterol: 106 mg | Sodium: 36 mg | Potassium: 139 mg | Phosphorus: 64 mg | Calcium: 36 mg | Fiber: 3g | Exchanges: ½ Starch, 1 Fruit, ½ Lean Meat | Gluten Free: Use gluten-free flour, vanilla, and cream of tartar

Baked Apples

This is a tasty way to use apples in the autumn, and is so much healthier than apple pie.

INGREDIENTS | SERVES 4

2 large apples, cored and cut in half

2 teaspoons lemon juice

4 packed teaspoons brown sugar

4 teaspoons oatmeal

Canola spray oil with butter flavor

⅛ cup water

1. Preheat oven to 375°F. Treat an ovenproof dish with nonstick cooking spray.

2. Place the apples cut-side up in the prepared dish and brush 1 teaspoon of the lemon juice over each apple.

3. In a small bowl, mix together the brown sugar and oatmeal and evenly divide over the apples. Mist the top of the apples with the spray oil. Add the water to the bottom of the baking dish.

4. Bake for 35 minutes, or until the apples are fork tender. Serve hot or cold.

PER SERVING: Calories: 79 | Protein: 0 g | Carbohydrates: 21 g | Fat: 0.2 g | Saturated Fat: 0 g | Cholesterol: 0 mg | Sodium: 3 mg | Potassium: 131 mg | Phosphorus: 15 mg | Calcium: 11 mg | Fiber: 3 g | Exchanges: 1½ Fruit | Gluten Free: Use gluten-free oatmeal

Grilled Pineapple

This is best cooked outdoors on a gas or charcoal grill.
Serve it with sugar-free ice cream or sorbet.

INGREDIENTS | SERVES 4

4 (¾") slices fresh pineapple, core and skin removed

2 teaspoons melted tub margarine (80% fat)

2 tablespoons no-calorie sweetener such as Splenda

Fruit on the Grill

Most fruits taste delicious grilled. With apples, peaches, pears, and apricots, it's best to leave the skins on and grill them flesh-side down.

1. Set your grill at medium-high, or wait until the coals turn white.

2. Brush both sides of the pineapple rings with margarine and sprinkle with sweetener.

3. Grill until you see grill marks, then turn. Grill for a few more minutes.

PER SERVING: Calories: 60 | Protein: 1 g | Carbohydrates: 12 g | Fat: 2 g | Saturated Fat:. 3 g | Cholesterol: 0 mg | Sodium: 16 mg | Potassium: 92 mg | Phosphorus: 7 mg | Calcium: 11 mg | Fiber: 1 g | Exchanges: ½ Fruit, ½ Fat | Gluten Free: Use gluten-free margarine

X Orange Carrot Cake

This delicious cake has a nice zing with the addition of a little lemon juice and the grated orange rind. The ginger root adds an appealing sophistication.

INGREDIENTS | SERVES 10

4 large eggs, separated
½ unpacked cup brown sugar
1½ cups grated carrots
1 tablespoon lemon juice
3 tablespoons freshly grated orange rind
½ cup corn flour
1" fresh ginger root, peeled and minced
1½ teaspoons baking soda
½ teaspoon salt

What's Up, Doc?

Carrot cake was created during World War II when flour and sugar were rationed. The sweetness of carrots contributed to this cake, and when oranges were available, it became a feast. Cooks used their fuel carefully, too, baking and making stews and soups in the oven all at the same time. Sometimes, hard times make for sweet endings.

1. Liberally spray canola spray oil on a a Springform pan and preheat oven to 325°F. Beat the egg whites until stiff and set aside.

2. Beat the egg yolks, sugar, and carrots together. Add lemon juice, orange rind, and corn flour. When smooth, add the ginger root, baking soda, and salt. Gently fold in the egg whites.

3. Pour the cake batter into the Springform pan and bake for 1 hour. Test by plunging a toothpick into the center of the cake—if the pick comes out clean, the cake is done.

PER SERVING: Calories: 86 | Protein: 3 g | Carbohydrates: 14 g | Fat: 2.1 g | Saturated Fat: 0.6 g | Cholesterol: 85 mg | Sodium: 340 mg | Potassium: 78 mg | Phosphorus: 46 mg | Calcium: 22 mg | Fiber: 1 g | Exchanges: 1 Starch | Gluten Free: Use gluten-free corn flour

⋋ Indian Pudding with Whipped Cream

*If you make too much, let it firm up, slice it, and fry the slices,
making sweet griddle cakes for breakfast the next day.*

INGREDIENTS | SERVES 8

4 cups 2% milk, divided
¼ cup white or yellow cornmeal
⅓ cup dark brown sugar
¼ cup white sugar
1 teaspoon salt
1 teaspoon cinnamon
¼ teaspoon ground nutmeg
1 teaspoon minced fresh ginger root
¼ cup molasses
5 teaspoons tub margarine (80% fat)

1. Preheat the oven to 250°F. Heat 2 cups milk.

2. Place the cornmeal and the rest of the dry ingredients, the ginger root, and molasses in the top of a double boiler.

3. Whisk the hot milk into the mixture, cooking and stirring over simmering water for 10 minutes, or until smooth.

4. Prepare a casserole dish with margarine. Whisk the cold milk into the hot mixture and pour into the baking dish.

5. Bake for 3 hours. Serve hot, or at room temperature with reduced-fat whipped cream, if desired.

PER SERVING: Calories: 174 | Protein: 4 g | Carbohydrates: 29 g | Fat: 5.0 g | Saturated Fat: 2.0 g | Cholesterol: 10 mg | Sodium: 374 mg | Potassium: 343 mg | Phosphorus: 125 mg | Calcium: 176 mg | Fiber: 1 g | Exchanges: 1 Starch, ½ Carbohydrate (count as Fruit), ½ Skim Milk, ½ Fat | Gluten Free: Use gluten-free margarine

Fruit Popsicles

If you don't have an ice crusher, place the ice in a plastic bag and smash it with a hammer or other hard object to crush it before adding it to a blender. The ice is important for bulking up the mixture.

INGREDIENTS | SERVES 6

1 (12-ounce) bag frozen unsweetened strawberries

3 cups 100% fruit strawberry juice

1 cup crushed ice

Homemade Popsicles

If you don't have a popsicle mold, don't fret. Just use paper cups! Allow the popsicles to freeze about 1 hour, then insert popsicle sticks or plastic spoons. Anything that stays in the center of the popsicle and makes a decent handle will work.

1. Place fruit, juice, and ice in a blender, in that order.

2. Blend on high.

3. Pour ingredients into popsicle molds.

4. Freeze for 1 hour. Remove popsicles from the freezer and insert a popsicle stick into the center of each treat. Return to the freezer and let solidify for another 7–9 hours before eating.

PER SERVING: Calories: 32 | Protein: 1 g | Carbohydrates: 8 g | Fat: 0.2 g | Saturated Fat: 0 g | Cholesterol: 0 mg | Sodium: 3 mg | Potassium: 150 mg | Phosphorus: 15 mg | Calcium: 16 mg | Fiber: 1 g | Exchanges: ½ Fruit | Gluten Free

Applesauce Sour Cream Coffee Cake

Add a peeled, chopped apple to the cake if you like.

INGREDIENTS | SERVES 20

1½ cups all-purpose flour

¾ cup packed light brown sugar (unpacked)

1 teaspoon baking soda

½ teaspoon low-sodium baking powder

1 teaspoon ground cinnamon

1 teaspoon salt

¾ cup fat-free sour cream

2 tablespoons canola oil

1 cup unsweetened applesauce

1. Preheat oven to 350°F.

2. Coat a square baking pan with light cooking spray.

3. Mix the flour, brown sugar, baking soda, baking powder, cinnamon, and salt in a large bowl.

4. Mix the sour cream, oil, and applesauce in a small bowl.

5. Add sour cream mixture to flour mixture. Mix well, but do not beat.

6. Pour batter into cake pan and bake until done, about 40 minutes.

PER SERVING: Calories: 80 | Protein: 1 g | Carbohydrates: 16 g | Fat: 1.5 g | Saturated Fat: 0.1 g | Cholesterol: 1 mg | Sodium: 195 mg | Potassium: 52 mg | Phosphorus: 29 mg | Calcium: 25 mg | Fiber: 1 g | Exchanges: 1 Starch | Gluten Free: Use gluten-free flour and baking powder

CHAPTER 19

Snacks and Beverages

Yogurt Fruit Smoothie

You can vary this smoothie by substituting other fruits of your choice. Good combinations are strawberry and banana, strawberry and kiwi, or banana and peach.

INGREDIENTS | SERVES 2

1 cup plain low-fat yogurt
½ cup fresh sliced strawberries
½ cup fresh orange juice
½ cup nectarines, peeled and sliced
2 tablespoons ground flax seed

Put all the ingredients in a blender and process until smooth.

PER SERVING: Calories: 170 | Protein: 9 g | Carbohydrates: 24 g | Fat: 5.2 g | Saturated Fat: 1.5 g | Cholesterol: 7 mg | Sodium: 89 mg | Potassium: 598 mg | Phosphorus: 250 mg | Calcium: 257 mg | Fiber: 3 g | Exchanges: 1¼ Fruit, ½ Skim Milk, ½ Lean Meat, ½ Fat | Gluten Free: Use gluten-free yogurt

Raspberry Almond Milk Frappe

The seeds in whole raspberries are a fabulous source of fiber. You can substitute maple syrup for honey in this recipe for a different flavor. You can also substitute other flavors of frozen yogurt to add variety.

INGREDIENTS | SERVES 2

1 cup unsweetened frozen raspberries
¾ cup vanilla frozen nonfat yogurt
½ cup almond milk (90 calories per cup)
⅛ teaspoon almond or vanilla extract

1. Place all the ingredients in a blender and blend until smooth.

2. Pour into 2 glasses and serve as a quick breakfast.

PER SERVING: Calories: 160 | Protein: 5 g | Carbohydrates: 33 g | Fat: 1.6 g | Saturated Fat: 0.1 g | Cholesterol: 1 mg | Sodium: 87 mg | Potassium: 377 mg | Phosphorus: 160 mg | Calcium: 206 mg | Fiber: 8 g | Exchanges: 1½ Fruit, ½ Skim Milk, ½ Fat | Gluten Free: Use gluten-free vanilla extract

Celery Peanut Butter Boats

Great for a picnic or potluck, these are a good way to get children to eat raw vegetables.

INGREDIENTS | SERVES 4

4 (5") ribs of celery, washed or wiped clean

4 teaspoons crunchy peanut butter

1 tablespoons toasted sesame seeds

1. Fill celery ribs with peanut butter and smooth out the top.

2. Cut the celery on the diagonal in to 1" slices.

3. Sprinkle the sesame seeds over the bites, and serve.

PER SERVING: Calories: 48 | Protein: 2 g | Carbohydrates: 2 g | Fat: 3.8 g | Saturated Fat: .6 g | Cholesterol: 0 mg | Sodium: 40 mg | Potassium: 93 mg | Phosphorus: 40 mg | Calcium: 12 mg | Fiber: 1 g | Exchanges: 1 Fat | Gluten Free: Use gluten-free peanut butter

Snacking with Celery

Crisp and spicy, celery is perfect with savory or slightly sweet fillings. Celery adds fiber to anything you pile into it, and its crunch is important in snacks. Fill it with light cream cheese and seeds or chopped toasted nuts. In a pinch, dip it in salad dressing. Fortunately, it's low in calories, and tastes wonderful.

Virgin Bellini

Try adding a drop of natural almond extract or food-grade peppermint oil to this delicious mocktail. Mint leaves make a pretty garnish.

INGREDIENTS | SERVES 4

2 large peaches, peeled, pitted, and cubed

1 tablespoon honey

Almond extract, to taste (optional)

Ice cubes, as needed

16 ounces seltzer water

1. In a blender or food processor, combine the peaches, honey, and almond extract, if using, and process until puréed.

2. Divide among 4 champagne flutes or tall glasses filled with ice cubes.

3. Add seltzer water, and stir. Serve immediately.

PER SERVING: Calories: 50 | Protein: 1 g | Carbohydrates: 13 g | Fat: 0.2 g | Saturated Fat: 0 g | Cholesterol: 0 mg | Sodium: 25 mg | Potassium: 171 mg | Phosphorus: 18 mg | Calcium: 12 mg | Fiber: 1 g | Exchanges: 1 Fruit | Gluten Free: Use gluten-free flavoring

Spiced Mixed Nut Butter

Serve Spiced Mixed Nut Butter with toast points, crackers, or celery sticks. Refrigerate any leftovers.

INGREDIENTS | SERVES 8

⅛ cup sesame seeds

⅛ cup dry roasted unsalted almonds, ground

⅛ cup sunflower seeds, hulled

½ tablespoon honey

¼ teaspoon cinnamon

⅛ teaspoon pumpkin pie spice

Pinch unsweetened cocoa powder

1. Bring a large, deep nonstick sauté pan to temperature over medium heat. Add the sesame seeds, ground almonds, and sunflower seeds and toast for 5–7 minutes, or until lightly browned, stirring frequently to prevent burning. Immediately transfer the nuts to a bowl, and let cool.

2. Combine the cooled, toasted nuts along with the remaining ingredients in a blender or food processor and process until the desired consistency is reached, scraping down the sides of the bowl as necessary. (Note: A mini food processor works best for a recipe this size.)

PER SERVING: Calories: 56 | Protein: 1 g | Carbohydrates: 6 g | Fat: 3.4 g | Saturated Fat: 0.3 g | Cholesterol: 0 mg | Sodium: 1 mg | Potassium: 43 mg | Phosphorus: 43 mg | Calcium: 12 mg | Fiber: 1 g | Exchanges: ⅓ Carbohydrate (count as Fruit), ⅔ Fat | Gluten Free

Kiwi Balls with Frosted Strawberries

Fixing a sweet and tasty icing for the berries makes a very pretty and delicious presentation.

INGREDIENTS | SERVES 4

1 tablespoon no-calorie sweetener such as Splenda

1 teaspoon cornstarch

½ teaspoon vanilla extract

1 teaspoon freshly squeezed lemon juice

1 tablespoon cold water

2 kiwi fruit, halved

12 medium-sized strawberries, hulled and halved

1. Whisk the sweetener, cornstarch, vanilla extract, lemon juice, and water together to make frosting. Set aside.

2. Use a melon ball scoop to make balls of the kiwi fruit. Put kiwis and strawberries in a bowl.

3. Take a heavy-duty plastic bag and cut a tiny piece from the corner. Spoon the frosting mixture into the bag and drizzle over the fruit.

4. Chill, and serve.

PER SERVING: Calories: 40 | Protein: 1 g | Carbohydrates: 9 g | Fat: 0.3 g | Saturated Fat: 0 g | Cholesterol: 0 mg | Sodium: 2 mg | Potassium: 176 mg | Phosphorus: 22 mg | Calcium: 19 mg | Fiber: 2 g | Exchanges: ½ Fruit | Gluten Free: Use gluten-free vanilla

Favorite Tools

Every kitchen needs two tiny implements—a melon ball scoop and a grapefruit spoon. The melon ball scoop is great for more than melon balls; it scoops up tiny tastes of all sorts of goodies. The grapefruit spoon has a sharp point and is excellent for cutting out the insides of tomatoes, avocados, potatoes, and many other foods.

Frozen Grapes

This snack is very sweet but not at all fattening.

INGREDIENTS | SERVES 8

1 pound seedless grapes, rinsed

2 teaspoons no-calorie sweetener such as Splenda

1 cup fat-free, sugar-free lemon yogurt

1. Prepare a cookie sheet with nonstick spray.

2. Place the damp grapes on the cookie sheet, sprinkle with sweetener, and freeze.

3. Use lemon yogurt as a dipping sauce for the frozen grapes.

PER SERVING: Calories: 68 | Protein: 2 g | Carbohydrates: 16 g | Fat: 0.3 g | Saturated Fat: 0.1 g | Cholesterol: 1 mg | Sodium: 19 mg | Potassium: 168 mg | Phosphorus: 42 mg | Calcium: 55 mg | Fiber: 1 g | Exchanges: 1 Fruit | Gluten Free: Use gluten-free yogurt

Chili Bean Dip with Dipping Vegetables

This is a great addition to any snack tray, whether for watching a game on TV or an after-school snack.

INGREDIENTS | SERVES 8

½ pound 80% lean ground beef

1 small onion, chopped

2 jalapeño peppers, cored, seeded, and chopped

2 cloves garlic, chopped

4 teaspoons chili powder, or to taste

1 (13-ounce) can crushed tomatoes with juice

1 (13-ounce) can red kidney beans

½ cup flat beer

1 cup each raw carrots, celery pieces, broccoli, spears of zucchini

1. Sauté the beef, onion, peppers, and garlic, breaking up with a spoon to avoid clumping.

2. When the vegetables are soft, drain fat and add chili powder, tomatoes, beans, and beer. Cover and simmer for 30 minute.

3. Let chili cool slightly, and pulse it in a food processor. Do not make it smooth. Serve alongside veggies.

PER SERVING: Calories: 137 | Protein: 8 g | Carbohydrates: 16 g | Fat: 5.0 g | Saturated Fat: 1.8 g | Cholesterol: 15 mg | Sodium: 253 mg | Potassium: 516 mg | Phosphorus: 122 mg | Calcium: 62 mg | Fiber: 5 g | Exchanges: ½ Starch, 2 Vegetable, 1 Lean Meat | Gluten Free: Use gluten-free beer and crushed canned tomatoes

Chili and Beans

There are endless variations of the chili-and-bean combination. Some people use turkey, others add dark chocolate and cinnamon and vary the amounts of beans and tomatoes. Some forms of chili don't have any beans. Various regions use various amounts of spice, heat, and ingredients.

Chunky Vegetable Dip

You can substitute onion soup mix for the vegetable soup mix.

INGREDIENTS | SERVES 10

1 large carrot
2 medium stalks celery
½ Vidalia onion
1 (8-ounce) carton fat-free sour cream
1 envelope vegetable soup mix
8 ounces unsalted potato chips

1. Boil the carrot, celery, and onion for 2–3 minutes.

2. Remove, drain, and cool the vegetables, then chop finely.

3. Mix the sour cream with the vegetable soup mix and add chopped vegetables.

4. Refrigerate the dip for at least 1 hour, and serve with chips.

PER SERVING: Calories: 158 | Protein: 3 g | Carbohydrates: 20 g | Fat: 8.1 g | Saturated Fat: 2.6 g | Cholesterol: 2 mg | Sodium: 308 mg | Potassium: 397 mg | Phosphorus: 72 mg | Calcium: 43 mg | Fiber: 2 g | Exchanges: 1 Starch, 1 Vegetable, 1½ Fat | Gluten Free: Use gluten-free vegetable soup mix and potato chips

Smoked Salmon Dip

*If you like a little kick in your dip, add a few dashes of Tabasco sauce to this recipe.
Serve with raw vegetables.*

INGREDIENTS | SERVES 4

1 cup fat-free sour cream
1 teaspoon lemon juice
½ teaspoon drained capers
1 small red onion, finely chopped
1 tablespoon unsalted tomato paste
¼ pound smoked salmon
Salt and pepper, to taste

Healthy Salmon

Salmon is low in calories and saturated fat, yet very high in protein. Salmon is an excellent source of omega-3 fatty acids, which can improve heart function and lower blood pressure. You can get omega-3 fatty acids from most cold-water fish, such as albacore tuna, salmon, and trout, which tend to have more of these good fats than other fish.

1. Mix all ingredients except the salmon and salt and pepper until well blended.

2. Chop the salmon into small pieces and mix it into the other ingredients.

3. Add the salt and pepper, to taste.

4. Refrigerate at least 1 hour before serving.

PER SERVING: Calories: 86 | Protein: 7 g | Carbohydrates: 11 g | Fat: 1.3 g | Saturated Fat: 0.3 g | Cholesterol: 12 mg | Sodium: 317 mg | Potassium: 190 mg | Phosphorus: 109 mg | Calcium: 80 mg | Fiber: 1 g | Exchanges: ¼ Skim Milk, 1 Lean Meat | Gluten Free: Use gluten-free tomato paste, salmon, and sour cream

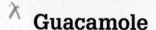

Guacamole

There are many recipes for guacamole. Some employ adobo sauce, others use tomatoes, and still others combine lemon and lime juice.

INGREDIENTS | SERVES 10

3 medium Hass avocados, peeled and seeded

Juice of 2 limes

½ cup finely minced sweet onion

1 teaspoon Tabasco sauce

½ teaspoon salt

2 tablespoons finely chopped fresh cilantro

1. Using a fork, mash the avocados.

2. Mix in the rest of the ingredients until well blended.

PER SERVING: Calories: 74 | Protein: 1 g | Carbohydrates: 5 g | Fat: 6.3 g | Saturated Fat: 0.9 g | Cholesterol: 0 mg | Sodium: 121 mg | Potassium: 237 mg | Phosphorus: 26 mg | Calcium: 9 mg | Fiber: 3 g | Exchanges: 1 Vegetable, 1 Fat | Gluten Free

Choosing Avocados

Most store-bought avocados are as hard as stones. That's fine; if you buy ripe ones, they generally have many blemishes. Just buy them a few days before you plan to serve them. Place them on a sunny windowsill or in a brown paper bag or wrap them in a newspaper; the paper seems to hasten ripening. The avocado should not have oily black spots in it when you cut it open but should be a uniform green. One or two black spots can be cut out, but don't use an avocado that is full of black spots or gray-brown areas.

Chickpea Parmesan Spread

This spread can be served hot or cold. Omit the hot sauce altogether if you have mild taste buds.

INGREDIENTS | SERVES 2

½ cup canned reduced-sodium chickpeas

2 tablespoons freshly grated Parmesan cheese

1 teaspoon olive oil

¼ teaspoon hot sauce

1. Drain and rinse the chickpeas. Mash chickpeas with a fork in a small bowl or mix in a blender until smooth.

2. Mix the Parmesan cheese with the chickpea mixture.

3. Add oil and hot sauce and blend well. Serve with pita bread crisps.

PER SERVING: Calories: 92 | Protein: 5 g | Carbohydrates: 10 g | Fat: 3.9 g | Saturated Fat: 1.2 g | Cholesterol: 4.4 mg | Sodium: 152 mg | Potassium: not enough to calculate | Phosphorus: not enough to calculate | Calcium: 76 mg | Fiber: 4 g | Exchanges: ½ Starch, ½ Lean Meat, ½ Fat | Gluten Free: Use gluten-free hot sauce

APPENDIX A

Meal Plans

A heart-healthy diet is needed for people with thyroid conditions. The recipes and meal plans in this book are designed to be included in most heart-healthy diets. A heart-healthy diet is one that is low in sodium and cholesterol, and you'll find this information listed with the recipes. Take advantage of the meal plans provided here, and use them to craft your own. Your medical team needs to be consulted, though, to make sure that the meal plans selected are appropriate.

Take Time to Plan

These meal plans are based on the diabetes exchange lists. The exchange lists have helped many people with diabetes (as well as those without diabetes) to lose and/or maintain weight. There are four meal plans offered with the following approximate caloric levels: 1,300 calories, 1,600 calories, 1,900 calories, and 2,200 calories.

Many women can maintain weight on 1,600–1,900 calories and lose weight on 1,300 calories. Women that are very small or inactive may need less, and extremely active women may need more. Many men can maintain weight on 1,900–2,200 calories and lose weight on approximately 1,600 calories. Websites such as USDA/ARS Children's Nutrition Research Center at Baylor College of Medicine (found at *www.bcm.edu/cnrc/caloriesneed.htm*) may be useful to help determine your individual caloric level. If your goal is to lose weight, it usually is recommended not to lose more than 1–2 pounds (2.2–4.4 kg) per week.

Remember, in order to lose weight, exercise should be a major part of your plan, if possible. Exercise helps burn calories, tone your body, and keep your heart fit! Ask your physician about how much exercise you need and can safely perform.

Follow these steps to plan your meals:

1. Ask your medical team what calorie level you need. You may use the government health sites to help you determine appropriate calorie levels.
2. Review Appendix B, and become familiar with this tool.
3. Select your favorite recipes from this book.
4. Plan meals using an appropriate number of exchanges in each food group for each meal and snack. (Exchanges in a heart-healthy diet include starch, fruit, skim milk, nonstarchy vegetables, lean meats and meat substitutes, and monounsaturated or polyunsaturated fat.) Plan at least 3–4 days of meals at once. If special conditions are needed, share your planned meals with your medical team. Use the plan to shop and stock your pantry; with the right foods available, making your meals will be easy.

You should spread out calories throughout the day, and eat breakfast, a snack, lunch, a snack, dinner, and a snack. It is usually alright to change the meal plan slightly and borrow exchanges from one meal or snack to use elsewhere in the day. With medical conditions such as type 1 diabetes, meals and snacks need to be consumed based on the type and time of insulin used. Consult your RD for advice and education.

On the following pages are sample plans for 1,300-, 1,600-, 1,900-, and 2,200-calorie diets.

1,300-Calorie Plan
52 percent calories from carbohydrate, 20 percent calories from protein, and 28 percent calories from fat.

FOOD GROUP	TOTAL NUMBER OF EXCHANGES	BREAKFAST	SNACK	LUNCH	SNACK	DINNER	SNACK
Starch	4	1		2		1	
Fruit	4	1	1		1		1
Skim Milk	2			1	1		
Vegetables	5	1		2		2	
Fats	3	1		1		1	

Meal Plan

BREAKFAST: 1 SERVING OF QUINOA BERRY BREAKFAST

1 Starch: Quinoa Berry Breakfast

1 Fruit: Quinoa Berry Breakfast (borrow ½ fruit from mid-morning snack)

1 Vegetable: Move to mid-morning snack

1 Lean Meat: ½ in quinoa berry breakfast, +½ ounce Canadian bacon

1 Fat: ½ in Quinoa Berry Breakfast, +2 extra walnut halves

SNACK: GRAPES AND NONSTARCHY VEGETABLES OF CHOICE

1 Fruit: ½ was consumed at breakfast +8 small grapes

1 Vegetable (moved from breakfast): 1 cup raw nonstarchy vegetables of choice

LUNCH: 1 SERVING OF EGGPLANT AND TOMATO STEW AND ½ CHICKEN SANDWICH

2 Starches: 1 in Eggplant and Tomato Stew, 1 ounce roll

1 Vegetables: 1 in Eggplant and Tomato Stew, 1 cup lettuce and tomato in sandwich

Lean Meat: 1 ounce chicken

1 Fat: ½ in Eggplant and Tomato Stew, ½ tablespoon salad dressing

SNACK: SMOOTHIE MADE WITH MILK, FRUIT, AND ICE

1 Fruit: 12 cherries

1 Skim Milk: 1 cup skim milk or 6–8 ounces skim milk yogurt

DINNER: 1 SERVING VEGETABLES IN WARM CITRUS VINAIGRETTE, CORN, SKIM MILK, RAW VEGETABLE SALAD, BROILED FISH OF CHOICE, PEANUTS, LOW-CALORIE SALAD DRESSING

1 Starch: ½ in Vegetables in Warm Citrus Vinaigrette, ¼ cup corn on salad

1 Skim Milk: 8 ounces skim milk

2 Vegetable: 1 in Vegetables in Warm Citrus Vinaigrette, 1 cup raw vegetables in salad

2 Lean Meat: 2 ounces broiled fish of choice

1 Fat: ½ in Vegetables in Warm Citrus Vinaigrette, ½ for 5 peanuts on salad

Free: 1 tablespoon low-calorie salad dressing

SNACK: CANTALOUPE

1 Fruit: 1 cup cantaloupe

1,600-Calorie Plan 58 percent carbohydrate, 20 percent protein, and 22 percent fat.

FOOD GROUP	TOTAL NUMBER OF EXCHANGES	BREAKFAST	SNACK	LUNCH	SNACK	DINNER	SNACK
Starch	6	1		2	1	2	
Fruit	5	1	1	1	1		1
Skim Milk	3			1		1	1
Vegetables	6	1	1	2		2	
Lean Meat	4	1		1		2	
Fats	4	1	1	1		1	

Meal Plan

BREAKFAST: 1 SERVING VEGETABLE OMELET, WHOLE-GRAIN BREAD, MELON, SUGAR-FREE JAM

1 Starch: 1 slice 80 calorie whole-grain bread of choice

1 Fruit: 1 cup mixed melon

1 Vegetable: In Vegetable Omelet

1 Lean Meat: In Vegetable Omelet, borrow ½ lean meat from lunch

1 Fat: 1 in Vegetable Omelet

Free: 2 teaspoons sugar-free jam

SNACK: BLACKBERRIES, NONSTARCHY VEGETABLES OF CHOICE, REDUCED-CALORIE SALAD DRESSING

1 Fruit: ¾ cup blackberries

1 Vegetable: 1 cup nonstarchy vegetables of choice

1 Fat: 2 tablespoons reduced-calorie salad dressing to dip vegetables in

LUNCH: 1 SERVING CHUNKY IRISH POTATO-LEEK SOUP, STRAWBERRIES AND BLUEBERRIES, SKIM MILK, RAW NONSTARCHY VEGETABLES FOR SALAD, LOW-FAT CHEESE, PEANUTS, LOW-CALORIE SALAD DRESSING

2 Starches: 3 starches in soup, borrow 1 from afternoon snack

1 Fruit: ¾–1 cup mixed strawberries and blueberries

1 Skim Milk: 1 cup skim milk

2 Vegetables: 1 in soup, 1 cup raw nonstarchy vegetables of choice for salad

1 Lean Meat: ½ borrowed from breakfast, ½ ounce low-fat cheese

1 Fat: ½ in soup, 10 peanuts on salad

Free: 1 tablespoon low-calorie salad dressing

SNACK: APPLE

1 Starch: Used at lunch

1 Fruit: 1 small apple

1,600-Calorie Meal Plan continued

DINNER: 1 SERVING FISH TACOS, RICE, SKIM MILK YOGURT, MIXED TOMATOES, SQUASH, AND MUSHROOMS, MARGARINE
2 Starches: 1 in Fish Tacos, ⅓ cup cooked rice
1 Skim milk: 6–8 ounces skim milk yogurt (less than 100 calories)
2 Vegetables: 1 in Fish Tacos, ½–1 cup cooked mixed tomatoes, squash, and mushrooms
2 Lean Meats: Both in Fish Tacos
1 Fat: ½ in Fish Tacos, ½ teaspoon margarine on vegetables
SNACK: DRIED CRANBERRIES, SKIM MILK YOGURT
1 Fruit: 2 tablespoons dried cranberries (no sugar added)
1 Skim Milk: 6–8 ounces skim milk yogurt (less than 100 calories)

1,900-Calorie Plan 57 percent carbohydrate, 20 percent protein, and 23 percent fat.

FOOD GROUP	TOTAL NUMBER OF EXCHANGES	BREAKFAST	SNACK	LUNCH	SNACK	DINNER	SNACK
Starch	8	2	1	2	1	2	
Fruit	6	1	1	1	1	1	1
Skim Milk	3					1	1
Vegetables	5	1				2	
Lean Meat	5	1				2	
Fats	5	1				2	1

Meal Plan

BREAKFAST: BUCKWHEAT PANCAKES, APPLESAUCE, TOMATO JUICE, EGG WHITES, MARGARINE
2 Starches: 1 serving Buckwheat Pancakes
1 Fruit: ½ cup applesauce
1 Vegetable: ½ cup tomato juice
1 Lean Meat: ½ save for lunch, ½ 1½ egg whites
1 Fat: 1 teaspoon margarine
SNACK: AIR POPPED POPCORN, PEACH
1 Starch: 3 cups air popped popcorn
1 Fruit: 1 medium peach

LUNCH: BAKED RED SNAPPER ALMANDINE, BANANA-BLUEBERRY OATMEAL BREAD, PLUM, PEAS, SKIM MILK, NONSTARCHY VEGETABLES FOR SALAD, BROCCOLI, MARGARINE

2 Starches: 1½ in bread, ¼ cup peas on salad

1 Fruit: ½ in bread, 1 plum

1 Skim Milk: 1 cup skim milk

2 Vegetables: 1 cup raw nonstarchy vegetables for salad, ½ cup cooked broccoli

2 Lean Meats: In the red snapper +½ lean meat saved from breakfast

1 Fat: 1 teaspoon margarine

SNACK: VIRGIN BELLINI, PRETZELS

1 Starch: ¾ ounce pretzels

1 Fruit: In Virgin Bellini

DINNER: WHOLE-WHEAT COUSCOUS SALAD, ROLL, WATERMELON, SKIM MILK, SIRLOIN STEAK, MARGARINE

2 Starches: ½ starch in couscous salad, 1½ ounce roll

1 Fruit: 1¼ cups watermelon

1 Skim Milk: 1 cup milk

2 Vegetables: In couscous salad

2 Lean Meats: 2 ounce sirloin steak

2 Fats: 1½ in couscous salad, 1½ teaspoons margarine

SNACK: CANNED PEARS, SKIM MILK YOGURT, ALMONDS

1 Fruit: ½ cup pears canned in juice

1 Skim milk: 6–8 ounces skim milk yogurt (less than 100 calories)

1 Fat: 6 almonds

2,200-Calorie Plan 56 percent carbohydrate, 20 percent protein, and 24 percent fat.

FOOD GROUP	TOTAL NUMBER OF EXCHANGES	BREAKFAST	SNACK	LUNCH	SNACK	DINNER	SNACK
Starch	10	3		3	1	2	1
Fruit	6	1	1	1	1	1	1
Skim Milk	3			1		1	1
Vegetables	7	1	1	2	1	2	
Lean Meat	6	1		2		3	
Fats	6	1	1	1	1	1	1

Meal Plan

BREAKFAST: CRANBERRY-CORNMEAL MUFFINS, COOKED CEREAL, BANANA, LOW-SODIUM VEGETABLE JUICE, EGG

3 Starches: 1 in muffin, +1 cup cooked cereal

1 Fruit: ¾ in muffin, + 1" of banana in cereal

1 Vegetable: ½ cup low-sodium vegetable juice

1 Lean Meat: 1 egg

1 Fat: In muffin

SNACK: KIWI, NONSTARCHY VEGETABLES, SALAD DRESSING

1 Fruit: 1 kiwi

1 Vegetable: 1 cup nonstarchy vegetables

1 Fat: 1 tablespoon salad dressing

LUNCH: 1 SERVING CHICKEN CORN CHOWDER, REDUCED-FAT CLUB CRACKERS, GINGERSNAPS, RASPBERRIES, SKIM MILK, RAW NONSTARCHY VEGETABLES, LOW FAT CHEESE, NUTS

3 Starches: 1 in chowder, 6 reduced fat club crackers, 3 gingersnaps

1 Fruit: 1 cup raspberries

1 Skim Milk: 1 cup skim milk

2 Vegetables: 1 in chowder, 1 cup raw nonstarchy vegetables

2 Lean Meats: 1½ in chowder, ½ ounce low-fat cheese

1 Fat: 1 tablespoon nuts (mixed with raspberries)

SNACK: REDUCED-FAT CLUB CRACKERS, PINEAPPLE, NONSTARCHY VEGETABLES, HAZELNUTS

1 Starch: Save ½ for dinner, 3 reduced fat club crackers

1 Fruit: ¾ cup raw pineapple

1 Vegetable: 1 cup nonstarchy vegetables

1 Fat: 5 hazelnuts

DINNER: BEEF RISOTTO, MANGO, SKIM MILK, NONSTARCHY VEGETABLES OVER LETTUCE, OYSTERS, DIET CHEESE

2 Starches: In risotto, + ½ starch from afternoon snack

1 Fruit: ½ mango

1 Skim Milk: 1 cup skim milk

2 Vegetables: 1½ in risotto, ¼ cup nonstarchy vegetables over lettuce

3 Lean Meats: 1 in risotto, 6 oysters, 1 ounce diet cheese (oysters and cheese can be for an appetizer)

1 Fat: In risotto

SNACK: GRAPENUTS, GRAPES, SKIM MILK YOGURT, CASHEWS

1 Starch: 3 tablespoons Grapenuts

1 Fruit: 15 grapes

1 Milk: 6–8 ounces skim milk yogurt (less than 100 calories)

1 Fat: 6 cashews

Exchange List

Because food exchange lists can be an important part of arriving at individualized meal plans, this appendix covers many of the common foods found on such lists. Please remember that the information contained in this book is not intended as medical advice. Consult your dietitian with any questions or details regarding the diet he or she has designed specifically for you. The information presented here is intended as a general guide only.

KEY

† = 3 grams or more of fiber per serving

‡ = High in sodium; if more than 1 serving is eaten, these foods have 400mg or more of sodium.

1 Carbohydrate Exchange List choice = 15 g carbohydrate

1 Protein Exchange List choice = 7 g protein

1 Milk Exchange List choice = 12 g carbohydrate and 8 g protein

1 Fat Exchange List choice = 5 g fat

Starches and Bread

These are the foods found on the bottom tier of the food pyramid. Each exchange in this category contains about 15 grams of carbohydrates, 3 grams of protein, and a trace of fat, for a total of 80 calories. Serving sizes may vary. A general rule is that ½ cup of cooked cereal, grain, or pasta equals 1 exchange, and 1 ounce of a bread product is 1 serving. Those foods within this category that contain 3 grams or more of fiber are identified using a † symbol.

BREAD	
food	**amount**
Plain roll, small	1 (1 ounce)
Raisin, unfrosted	1 slice
Rye†, pumpernickel	1 slice (1 ounce)
Tortilla, 6" across	1
White (including French, Italian)	1 slice (1 ounce)
Whole wheat	1 slice
CEREALS AND PASTA	
Bran cereals†, concentrated	
100 percent Bran	⅔ cup
All Bran	⅓ cup
All-Bran with extra fiber	1 cup
Bran Buds	⅓ cup
Bran Chex	½ cup
Fiber One	⅔ cup
Multi-Bran Chex	⅓ cup

Bran cereals†, flaked	
40 percent bran flakes	½ cup
Fortified Oat Flakes	⅓ cup
Nutri-Grain	½ cup
Bulgur, cooked	½ cup
CEREALS, MOST READY TO EAT,	
unsweetened, plain	¾ cup
Cheerios†	1 cup
Cooked cereals	½ cup
Cornflakes	¾ cup
Frosted Flakes	¼ cup
Grape Nuts	3 tablespoons
Grits, cooked	½ cup
Kix	1 cup
Life	½ cup
Puffed cereal, rice or wheat	1½ cups
Rice Krispies	⅔ cup
Shredded wheat, biscuit	1 cup
Shredded wheat, spoon size	½ cup
Shredded Wheat and Bran†	½ cup
Special K	1 cup
Total	¾ cup
Wheat Chex†	½ cup
Wheaties†	⅔ cup
GRAINS	
Barley, cooked	⅓ cup
Buckwheat, cooked	½ cup
Bulgur, cooked	⅓ cup
Cornmeal, dry	2½ tablespoons
Cornstarch	2 tablespoons
Couscous, cooked	⅓ cup
Flour	3 tablespoons
Kasha, cooked	⅓ cup
Millet, dry	3 tablespoons
Oat bran, cooked	¼ cup
Pasta, cooked	⅓ cup
Quinoa, cooked	⅓ cup
Rice, white or brown, cooked	⅓ cup

GRAINS	
Rice, wild, cooked	½ cup
Wheat berries, cooked	⅔ cup
Wheat germ†	¼ cup
(1 carb and 1 low-fat protein) CRACKERS AND SNACKS	
Animal crackers	8
Cheese Nips, reduced fat	22
Club, reduced fat	6
Finn Crisp	4
Graham crackers, (2½" square)	3
Matzoh	1 (¾ ounce)
Matzoh with bran	1 (¾ ounce)
Manischewitz whole-wheat matzoh crackers	7
Melba toast, rectangles	5
Melba toast, rounds	10
Mr. Phipps pretzel chips‡	12
Orville Redenbacher Smart Pop! popcorn	3 cups
Popcorn, air popped, no fat added	3 cups
Pretzels‡	¾ ounce
Rye crisp, 2" × 3½"	4
Saltine-type crackers‡	6
Snack-Well's, fat-free, cheddar‡	24
Snack-Well's, fat-free, cracked pepper	8
Snack-Well's, fat-free, wheat	6
Town House, reduced fat‡	8
Triscuits, reduced fat‡	8
Wasa Golden Rye	2
Wasa Hearty Rye	2
Wasa Lite	2
DRIED BEANS, LENTILS, AND PEAS Note: All portions given are for cooked amounts.	
Baked beans†	⅓ cup
Beans†, white	½ cup
Chickpeas/Garbanzo beans†	½ cup
Kidney beans†	½ cup
Lentils†	½ cup
Lima beans†	⅔ cup

DRIED BEANS, LENTILS, AND PEAS	
Navy beans†	½ cup
Peas†, black-eyed	½ cup
Peas†, split	½ cup
Pinto beans†	½ cup
STARCHY VEGETABLES	
Corn†	½ cup
Corn on the cob†, 6" long	1
Lima beans†	½ cup
Mixed vegetables, with corn or peas	⅔ cup
Peas†, green (canned or frozen)	½ cup
Plantain†	½ cup
Potato, baked or boiled	1 small (3 ounce)
Potato, mashed	½ cup
Pumpkin	1 cup
Squash, winter (acorn, butternut)	1 cup
Yam, sweet potato	½ cup
STARCHES AND BREADS PREPARED WITH FAT These count as 1 starch/bread plus 1 fat choice	
Biscuit, 2½" across	1
Chow mein noodles	½ cup
Corn bread, 2" cube	1 (2 ounce)
Crackers:	
Arrowroot	4
Butter cracker‡, round	7
Butter cracker‡, rectangle	6
Cheese Nips‡	20
Cheez-It‡	27
Club‡	6
Combos‡	1 ounce
Escort‡	5
Lorna Doone	3
Meal Mates‡	5
Oyster‡	20
Peanut butter crackers‡	3
Pepperidge Farm Bordeaux cookies	3
Pepperidge Farm Goldfish‡	36
Popcorn, microwave, light	4 cups

STARCHES AND BREADS PREPARED WITH FAT	
Ritz‡	7
Sociables‡	9
Stella D'oro Sesame Breadsticks	2
Sunshine HiHo‡	6
Teddy Grahams	15
Tidbits‡	21
Triscuits‡	5
Town House‡	6
Vanilla Wafers	6
Wasa Breakfast crispbread	2
Wasa Fiber Plus crispbread	4
Wasa Sesame crispbread	2
Waverly Wafers‡	2
Wheat Thins, reduced fat‡	13
French fries (2" to 3" long)	10 (1½ ounces)
Muffin, plain, small	1
Pancake, 4" across	2
Stuffing, bread (prepared)	¼ cup
Taco shell, 6" across	2
Waffle, 4½" square	1

Vegetables

Vegetables fall within the second tier of the food pyramid. Each vegetable serving is calculated to contain 5 grams of carbohydrates, 2 grams of protein, between 2 to 3 grams of fiber, and 25 calories. Vegetables are a good source of vitamins and minerals. Fresh or frozen vegetables are preferred because of their higher vitamin and mineral content; however, canned vegetables are also acceptable, with the preference being for low-sodium or salt-free varieties. As a general rule, one Vegetable Exchange is usually equal to ½ cup cooked, 1 cup raw, or ½ cup juice.

Not all vegetables are found on the Vegetable Exchange List. Starchy vegetables such as corn, peas, and potatoes are part of the Starches and Bread Exchange List. Vegetables with fewer than 10 calories per serving are found on the Free Food Exchange List.

VEGETABLE EXCHANGE LIST Cooked or steamed serving.			
Artichoke	½ medium	Okra	½ cup
Asparagus	1 cup	Onions	½ cup
Bamboo shoots	1 cup	Pea pods	½ cup
Bean sprouts	½ cup	Radishes	1 cup
Beet greens	½ cup	Red pepper	1 cup
Beets	½ cup	Rutabaga	½ cup
Broccoli	½ cup	Sauerkraut‡	½ cup
Brussels sprouts	½ cup	Spaghetti sauce, jar	¼ cup
Cabbage	1 cup	Spaghetti squash	½ cup
Carrots	½ cup	Spinach	½ cup
Cauliflower	½ cup	Summer squash	1 cup
Celery	1 cup	Tomato	1 medium
Collard greens	1 cup	Tomato, canned‡	½ cup
Eggplant	½ cup	Tomato, paste‡	1½ tablespoons
Fennel leaf	1 cup	Tomato sauce, canned‡	⅓ cup
Green beans	1 cup	Tomato/vegetable juice‡	½ cup
Green pepper	1 cup	Turnip greens	1 cup
Kale	½ cup	Turnips	½ cup
Kohlrabi	½ cup	Water chestnuts	6 whole or ½ cup
Leeks	½ cup	Wax beans	½ cup
Mushrooms, fresh	1 cup	Zucchini	1 cup
Mustard greens	1 cup		

Fruits

One Fruit Exchange has about 15 grams of carbohydrates, which totals 60 calories. The serving sizes for fruits vary considerably, so consult the list. Also, note that portion amounts are given for fruit that is dried, fresh, frozen, or canned packed in its own juice with no sugar added.

FRESH, FROZEN, AND UNSWEETENED CANNED FRUIT	
Apple, raw, 2" across	1
Apple, dried	4 rings
Applesauce, unsweetened	½ cup
Apricots, canned	4 halves or ½ cup

FRESH, FROZEN, AND UNSWEETENED CANNED FRUIT	
Apricots, dried	8 halves
Apricots, fresh, medium	4
Banana, 9" long	½
Banana flakes or chips	3 tablespoons
Blackberries, raw	¾ cup
Blueberries†, raw	¾ cup
Boysenberries	1 cup
Canned fruit, unless otherwise stated	½ cup
Cantaloupe, 5" across	⅓
Cantaloupe, cubes	1 cup
Casaba, 7" across	⅙ melon
Casaba, cubed	1⅓ cups
Cherries, large, raw	12 whole
Cherries, canned	½ cup
Cherries, dried (no sugar added)	2 tablespoons
Cranberries, dried (no sugar added)	2 tablespoons
Currants	2 tablespoons
Dates	3
Fig, dried	1
Figs, fresh, 2" across	2
Fruit cocktail, canned	½ cup
Grapefruit, medium	½
Grapefruit, sections	¾ cup
Grapes, small	15
Guavas, small	1½
Honeydew melon, medium	⅛
Honeydew melon, cubes	1 cup
Kiwi, large	1
Kumquats, medium	5
Loquats, fresh	12
Lychees, dried or fresh	10
Mandarin oranges	¾ cup
Mango, small	½
Nectarine, 2½" across	1
Orange, 3" across	1
Papaya, fresh, 3½" across	½
Papaya, fresh, cubed	1 cup
Peach, 2¾" across	1 peach or ¾ cup

FRESH, FROZEN, AND UNSWEETENED CANNED FRUIT	
Peaches, canned	2 halves or 1 cup
Peach, fresh, 2½" across	1
Pear, small	1
Pears, canned	2 halves or ½ cup
Persimmon, medium, native	2
Pineapple, raw	¾ cup
Pineapple, canned	⅓ cup
Plantain, cooked	⅓ cup
Plum, raw, 2" across	2
Pomegranate†	½
Prunes, dried, medium	3
Raisins	2 tablespoons
Raspberries†, raw	1 cup
Strawberries†, raw, whole	1¼ cups
Tangerine, 2½" across	2
Watermelon, cubes	1¼ cups
DRIED FRUIT†	
Apples †	4 rings
Apricots †	8 halves
Dates, medium	2½
Figs †	1½
Prunes, medium †	3
Raisins	2 tablespoons
FRUIT JUICE	
Apple cider	½ cup
Apple juice, unsweetened	½ cup
Cranapple juice, unsweetened	⅜ cup
Cranberry juice cocktail	⅓ cup
Cranberry juice, low-calorie	1⅛ cups
Cranberry juice, unsweetened	½ cup
Grapefruit juice	½ cup
Grape juice	⅓ cup
Orange juice	½ cup
Pineapple juice	½ cup
Prune juice	⅓ cup

Milk

Milk servings are usually marked at 1 cup or 8 ounces. Like meats, Milk Exchange Lists are divided into categories depending on the fat content of the choices. Each Milk Exchange has about 12 grams of carbohydrate and 8 grams of protein; however, the calories in each exchange will vary according to the fat content.

SKIM OR VERY LOW-FAT MILK	
½% milk	1 cup
1% milk	1 cup
Buttermilk, low-fat or 1%	1 cup
Nonfat milk, dry	⅓ cup
Skim milk	1 cup
Skim milk, evaporated	½ cup
Yogurt, plain, nonfat	8 ounces
LOW-FAT MILK	
2% milk	1 cup
Yogurt, plain, low-fat with added nonfat milk solids	8 ounces
WHOLE MILK	
Whole milk	1 cup
Whole milk, evaporated	½ cup
Yogurt, plain, whole milk	8 ounces

The whole-milk group has much more fat per serving than the skim and low-fat groups. Whole milk has more than 3¼ percent butterfat, so you should limit your choices from this group as much as possible.

Meats

Each serving of meat or meat substitute has about 7 grams of protein. As shown in the tables below, the Meats Exchange Lists are divided depending on the fat content of the meat or meat substitute choice. (See Chapter 5 for suggestions on the healthiest ways to prepare meats.)

Make your selections from the lean and medium-fat meat, poultry, and fish choices in your meal plan as much as possible. This helps you keep the fat intake in your diet low, which may help decrease your risk for heart disease. Remember that the meats in the high-fat group have more saturated fat, cholesterol, and calories, so you should consult with your dietitian about whether or not your diet should include any meats from that group. When they are permitted, most dieticians recommend limiting your choices from the high-fat group to a maximum of three times per week.

Meats and meat substitutes that have 400 milligrams or more of sodium per exchange are indicated with the ‡ symbol.

Meats Exchange List portions are generally 1 ounce of cooked meat (using the 4 ounces of raw meat results in 3 ounces of cooked meat standard). Beef, pork, fish, poultry, cheese, eggs, and, when they're used as meat substitutes, dried beans, legumes, and some nuts, fall within the Meats Exchange Lists categories. Because the calorie counts vary so widely (as does the cholesterol and saturated fat content), your dietician will advise from which lists you are to choose your selections.

exchange	carbohydrate	protein (g)	fat(g)	calories
Very-Lean Meats	0	7	0–1	35
Lean Meats	0	7	3	55
Medium-Fat	0	7	5	75
High-Fat	0	7	8	100

VERY-LEAN MEATS (AND MEAT SUBSTITUTES)

Meats in this category are usually the reduced-fat varieties, like Healthy Choice, and contain 4 percent or fewer calories from fat, which unless otherwise noted below are at 1 ounce per Food Exchange List portion. Name-brand foods come and go, with new ones introduced regularly that phase out others. Check product labels or with your dietician to ascertain which products currently fall within this category.
One choice provides about 35–45 calories, 7 grams of protein, no carbohydrates, and 0–2 grams of fat.

Buffalo	1 ounce
Chicken, white meat, skinless	1 ounce
Cornish hen, white meat, skinless	1 ounce
Cottage cheese, fat free or 1%	¼ cup
Ricotta, 100 percent fat free‡	1 ounce
Egg substitute, plain (if less than 40 calories per serving)	¼ cup

VERY-LEAN MEATS (AND MEAT SUBSTITUTES)	
Fish and seafood, fresh or frozen, cooked: clams, cod, crab, flounder, haddock, halibut, imitation crabmeat, lobster, scallops, shrimp, trout, tuna (in water)	2 ounces
Ostrich	1 ounce
Turkey, ground, 93–99 percent fat free	1 ounce
Turkey, white meat, skinless	1 ounce
Turkey sausage, 97 percent fat free‡	1 ounce
Venison	1 ounce
LEAN MEATS (AND MEAT SUBSTITUTES) One choice provides about 55 calories, 7 grams of protein, no carbohydrates, and 3 grams of fat.	
95 percent fat-free luncheon meat	1 ounce
Beef, of lean beef such as:	
Chipped beef‡ (USDA Good or Choice grade)	1 ounce
Flank steak (USDA Good or Choice grade)	1 ounce
Round steak (USDA Good or Choice grade)	1 ounce
Sirloin steak (USDA Good or Choice grade)	1 ounce
Tenderloin (USDA Good or Choice grade)	1 ounce
Clams, fresh or canned in water‡	2 ounces
Cottage cheese, any variety	¼ cup
Crab	2 ounces
Diet cheese‡ (with fewer than 55 calories per ounce)	1 ounce
Duck, without skin	1 ounce
Egg substitutes (with fewer than 55 calories per ¼ cup)	¼ cup
Egg whites	3
Fish, all fresh and frozen catfish, salmon, and other fattier fish	1 ounce
Goose, without skin	1 ounce
Grated Parmesan	2 tablespoons
Herring, uncreamed or smoked	1 ounce
Lobster	2 ounces
Oysters, medium	6
Pheasant, without skin	1 ounce
Boiled ham‡	1 ounce
Canadian bacon‡	1 ounce
Canned ham‡	1 ounce
Cured ham‡	1 ounce
Fresh ham	1 ounce
Tenderloin	1 ounce
Chicken, dark meat, without skin	1 ounce

LEAN MEATS (AND MEAT SUBSTITUTES)	
Cornish game hen, dark meat, without skin	1 ounce
Turkey, dark meat, without skin	1 ounce
Rabbit	1 ounce
Sardines, canned, medium	2
Scallops	2 ounces
Shrimp	2 ounces
Squirrel	1 ounce
Tofu	3 ounces
Veal, all cuts are lean except for veal cutlets (ground or cubed)	1 ounce
Venison	1 ounce
MEDIUM-FAT MEATS (AND MEAT SUBSTITUTES) One choice provides about 75 calories, 7 grams of protein, no carbohydrates, and 5 grams of fat.	
86 percent fat-free luncheon meat‡	1 ounce
Chuck roast	1 ounce
Cubed steak	1 ounce
Ground beef	1 ounce
Meat loaf	1 ounce
Porterhouse steak	1 ounce
Rib roast	1 ounce
Rump roast	1 ounce
T-bone steak	1 ounce
Diet cheeses‡ (with 56–80 calories per ounce)	1 ounce
Mozzarella (skim or part-skim milk)	1 ounce
Ricotta (skim or part-skim milk)	¼ cup
Egg (high in cholesterol, so limit to 3 per week)	1
Egg substitutes (with 56–80 calories per ¼ cup)	¼ cup
Heart (high in cholesterol)	1 ounce
Kidney (high in cholesterol)	1 ounce
Lamb chops	1 ounce
Lamb leg	1 ounce
Lamb roast	1 ounce
Liver (high in cholesterol)	1 ounce
Parmesan cheese‡	3 tablespoons
Pork chops	1 ounce
Pork loin roast	1 ounce
Boston butt	1 ounce
Pork cutlets	1 ounce

MEDIUM-FAT MEATS (AND MEAT SUBSTITUTES)	
Chicken (with skin)	1 ounce
Duck, domestic, well drained of fat	1 ounce
Goose, domestic, well drained of fat	1 ounce
Ground turkey	1 ounce
Romano cheese	3 tablespoons
Sweetbreads (high in cholesterol)	1 ounce
Tofu (2½" × 2¾" × 1")	4 ounce
Tuna‡, canned in oil, drained	¼ cup
Salmon‡, canned	¼ cup
Veal cutlet, ground or cubed, unbreaded	1 ounce
HIGH-FAT MEATS (AND MEAT SUBSTITUTES) Remember, these items are high in saturated fat, cholesterol, and calories, and should be eaten only three or fewer times per week. One choice provides about 100 calories, 7 grams of protein, no carbohydrates, and 8 grams of fat. One exchange choice is equal to any one of the following items:	
Most USDA Prime cuts of beef	1 ounce
Beef‡, corned	1 ounce
Ribs, beef	1 ounce
Bologna‡	1 ounce
Cheese, all regular cheese‡:	
American	1 ounce
Bleu	1 ounce
Cheddar	1 ounce
Monterey	1 ounce
Swiss	1 ounce
Fish, fried	1 ounce
Hotdog‡:	
Chicken, 10/pound	1 frank
Turkey, 10/pound	1 frank
Lamb, ground	1 ounce
Peanut butter (contains unsaturated fat)	1 tablespoon
Pimiento loaf‡	1 ounce
Pork chop	1 ounce
Pork, ground	1 ounce
Spareribs	1 ounce
Steak	1 ounce
Salami‡	1 ounce

Sausage‡:	
Bratwurst‡	1 ounce
Italian	1 ounce
Knockwurst, smoked	1 ounce
Polish	1 ounce
Pork sausage‡ (patty or link)	1 ounce
Counts as one high-fat meat *plus* one fat exchange:	
Hotdog‡—beef, pork, or combination, 400mg or more of sodium per exchange, 10/pound	1 frank

Fats

Each Fats Exchange List serving will contain about 5 grams of fat and 45 calories. Fats are found in margarine, butter, oils, nuts, meat fat, and dairy products. Saturated fat amounts and sodium contents can vary considerably, depending on the choice. Most dieticians recommend polyunsaturated or monounsaturated fats whenever possible.

UNSATURATED FATS	
Almonds, dry roasted	6
Avocado, medium	⅛
Cashews, dry roasted	1 tablespoon or 6
Cooking oil (corn, cottonseed, safflower, soybean, sunflower, olive, peanut)	1 teaspoon
Hazelnuts (filberts)	5
Macadamia nuts	3
Margarine	1 teaspoon
Margarine, diet‡	1 tablespoon
Mayonnaise	1 teaspoon
Mayonnaise, reduced calorie‡	1 tablespoon
Olives, black, large‡	9
Olives, green, large‡	10
Other nuts	1 tablespoon
Peanuts, large	10
Peanuts, small	20
Pecan halves	4
Pine nuts	1 tablespoon

UNSATURATED FATS	
Pistachio	12
Pumpkin seeds	2 teaspoons
Salad dressing, all varieties, regular	1 tablespoon
Salad dressing, mayonnaise-type, reduced calorie	1 tablespoon
Salad dressing, mayonnaise-type, regular	2 teaspoons
Salad dressing, reduced calorie‡ (2 tablespoons of low-calorie dressing is a free food)	2 tablespoons
Sesame seeds	1 tablespoon
Sunflower seeds, without shells	1 tablespoon
Tahini	2 teaspoons
Walnut halves	4
SATURATED FATS	
Bacon‡	1 slice
Butter	1 teaspoon
Butter, whipped	2 teaspoons
Chitterlings	½ ounce
Coconut, shredded	2 tablespoons
Coffee whitener, liquid	2 tablespoons
Coffee whitener, powder	4 tablespoons
Cream, heavy	1 tablespoon
Cream, light, coffee, table	2 tablespoons
Cream, sour	2 tablespoons
Cream, whipping	1 tablespoon
Cream cheese	1 tablespoon
Salt pork‡	¼ ounce

Free Foods

A free food is any food or drink that contains fewer than 20 calories per serving. Unless a serving size is specified, you can eat as much as you want of these foods. You are limited to eating two or three servings per day of those foods with a specific serving size.

FREE DRINKS	
Bouillon or canned broth without fat‡	
Bouillon, low sodium	
Broth, low sodium	
Carbonated drinks, sugar free	
Carbonated water	
Club soda	
Cocoa powder, unsweetened	1 tablespoon
Coffee	
Drink mixes, sugar free	
Tea	
Tonic water, sugar free	
FREE FRUITS AND VEGETABLES	
Cranberries, unsweetened	½ cup
Rhubarb, unsweetened	½ cup
Vegetables, raw	1 cup
Alfalfa sprouts	
Cabbage	
Celery	
Chinese cabbage†	
Cucumber	
Endive	
Escarole	
Green onion	
Hot peppers	
Lettuce	
Mushrooms	
Parsley	
Pickles, unsweetened‡	
Pimento	
Radishes	
Romaine	
Salad greens	
Spinach	
Watercress	
Zucchini†	

FREE SWEETS	
Candy, hard, sugar free	
Gelatin, sugar free	
Gum, sugar free	
Jam/jelly, low sugar	2 teaspoons
Jam/jelly, sugar free	2 teaspoons
Pancake syrup, sugar free	1–2 tablespoons
Sugar substitutes (saccharin, aspartame, Splenda)	
Whipped topping	2 tablespoons
FREE CONDIMENTS	
Horseradish	
Ketchup	1 tablespoon
Mustard	
Nonstick pan spray	
Pickles, dill, unsweetened‡	
Salad dressing, low calorie	2 tablespoons
Taco sauce	1 tablespoon
Vinegar	
FREE SEASONINGS Seasonings can be very helpful in making foods taste better, but be careful how much sodium you use. Read labels to help you choose seasonings that do not contain sodium or salt.	
Basil	
Celery seeds	
Chili powder	
Chives	
Cinnamon	
Curry	
Dill	
Garlic	
Garlic powder	
Herbs	
Hot pepper sauce	
Lemon	
Lemon juice	
Lemon pepper	
Lime	
Lime juice	

FREE SEASONINGS	
Mint	
Onion powder	
Oregano	
Paprika	
Pepper	
Pimiento	
Soy sauce, low sodium ("lite")	
Soy sauce‡	
Spices	
Wine, used in cooking	¼ cup
Worcestershire sauce‡	
FREE FLAVORING EXTRACTS	
Almond	
Butter	
Lemon	
Peppermint	
Vanilla	
Walnut	

MEAT SUBSTITUTE PROTEIN FOODS Note: Foods on this list equal 1 Protein Food Exchange List serving (0g carb, 7g protein, 0–5 gfat).	
Egg substitute	¼ cup
Soy cheese	1 ounce
Tofu, firm	½ cup (4 ounces)

BEANS USED AS A MEAT SUBSTITUTE		
Dried beans†	1 cup, cooked	1 lean meat, 2 starches
Dried lentils†	1 cup, cooked	1 lean meat, 2 starches
Dried peas†	1 cup, cooked	1 lean meat, 2 starches

NUTS AND SEEDS USED AS A MEAT SUBSTITUTE	
Note: Foods on this list equal 1 Protein and 2 or 3 Fat Food Exchange List serving (0g carb, 7g protein, 10–15g fat). Consult product label to determine fat content for your choice.	
Almonds	¼ cup
Pecans	¼ cup
Peanuts	¼ cup
Pine nuts	2 tablespoons
Pistachios	¼ cup (1 ounce)
Pumpkin seeds	¼ cup
Sesame seeds	¼ cup
Squash seeds	¼ cup
Sunflower seeds	¼ cup
Walnut halves	16–20

Combination Foods

Food is often mixed together in various combinations that do not fit into only one exchange list. Each of the recipes in this book gives the exchange list exchanges for that dish. The following is included as a list of average exchange list values for some typical combination foods. Ask your dietitian for information about these or any other combination of foods you'd like to eat.

FAT FOODS USED AS A MEAT SUBSTITUTE		
Note: Foods on this list equal 1 Fat Food Exchange List serving(0g carb, 5g fat).		
Almond butter	1 tablespoon	2 fats
Cashew butter	1 tablespoon	2 fats
Flax seed oil	1 teaspoon	1 fat
Peanut oil	1 teaspoon	1 fat
Sesame butter	1 tablespoon	2 fats

Foods for Special Treats

These foods, despite their sugar or fat content, are intended to be added to your meal plan in moderate amounts, as long as your dietitian agrees and if, despite consuming them, you can still maintain blood-glucose control. Your dietitian can also advise how often you can eat these foods. Because these special treats are concentrated sources of carbohydrate, the portion sizes are small.

COMBO FOODS		
Bean soup†‡	1 cup (8 ounces)	1 lean meat, 1 starch, 1 vegetable
Casserole		2 medium-fat meats
Homemade Casserole	1 cup (8 ounces)	2 starches, 1 fat
Cheese pizza‡, thin crust	¼ of 15-ounce pizza	1 medium-fat meat
Cheese pizza‡, 10" pizza		2 starches, 1 fat
Chili with beans, commercial†‡	1 cup (8 ounces)	2 medium-fat meats, 2 starches, 2 fats
Chow mein†‡ (without noodles or rice)	2 cups (16 ounces)	2 lean meats, 1 starch, 2 vegetables
Chunky soup, all varieties‡	10¾-ounce can	1 medium-fat meat, 1 starch, 1 vegetable
Cream soup‡ (made with water)	1 cup (8 ounces)	1 starch, 1 fat
Macaroni and cheese‡	1 cup (8 ounces)	1 medium-fat meat, 2 starches, 2 fats
Spaghetti and meatballs, canned‡	1 cup (8 ounces)	1 medium-fat meat, 1 fat, 2 starches
Sugar-free pudding (made with skim milk)	½ cup	1 starch
Vegetable soup‡	1 cup (8 ounces)	1 starch

FOODS FOR SPECIAL TREATS		
Angel-food cake	1/12 cake	2 starches
Cake, no icing	1/12 cake (3" square)	2 starches, 2 fats
Cookies	2 small (1¾" across)	2 starches, 1 fat
Frozen fruit yogurt	⅓ cup	1 starch
Gingersnaps	3	1 starch
Granola	¼ cup	1 starch, 1 fat
Granola bars	1 small	1 starch, 1 fat
Ice cream, any flavor	½ cup	1 starch, 2 fats
Ice milk, any flavor	½ cup	1 starch, 1 fat
Sherbet, any flavor	¼ cup	1 starch
Snack chips‡, all varieties	1 ounce	1 starch, 2 fats
Vanilla wafers	6 small	1 starch, 2 fats

MISCELLANEOUS FOODS				
Jam, regular	1 tablespoon	1 carbohydrate	13g	80
Jelly, regular	1 tablespoon	1 carbohydrate	13g	80
Honey, regular	1 tablespoon	1 carbohydrate	13g	80
Sugar	1 tablespoon	1 carbohydrate	12g	46
Syrup, light	2 tablespoons	1 carbohydrates	13g	80
Syrup, regular	2 tablespoons	2 carbohydrates	27g	160
Yogurt, regular, with fruit	1 cup	3 carbohydrates	45g	240

OTHER SPECIAL FOODS		
Brewer's yeast	3 tablespoons	1 bread
Carob flour	⅛ cup	1 bread
Kefir	1 cup	1 milk, 1 fat
Miso	3 tablespoons	1 bread, ½ lean meat
Sea vegetables, cooked	½ cup	1 vegetable
Soy flour	¼ cup	1 lean meat, ½ bread
Soy grits, raw	⅛ cup	1 lean meat
Soy milk	1 cup	1 milk, 1 fat
Tahini	1 teaspoon	1 fat
Tempeh	4 ounces	1 bread, 2 protein
Wheat germ	1 tablespoon	½ bread

Measuring Foods

Portion control is an important part of implementing a diet based on the Food Exchange Lists. This helps ensure you eat the right serving sizes of food. Liquids and some solid foods (such as tuna, cottage cheese, and canned fruits) can be measured using a measuring cup. Measuring spoons are useful to guarantee correct amounts for foods used in smaller portions, like oil, salad dressing, and peanut butter. A scale can be very useful for measuring almost anything, especially meat, poultry, and fish.

Similar in manner to how professional chefs cook, you will eventually learn how to estimate food amounts. Until then, it can be useful to remember that 1 cup is about equal in size to an average woman's closed fist. A thumb is about the size of 1 tablespoon or a 1-ounce portion of cheese. The tip of the thumb equals about 1 teaspoon, a useful gauge when trying to determine how much butter to add to your bread or dressing to add to a salad when you're dining out and don't have measuring spoons available.

Many raw foods will weigh less after they are cooked. This is especially true for most meats. On the other hand, starches often swell during cooking, so a small amount of uncooked starch results in a much larger amount of cooked food. Some examples of those changes are:

STARCH GROUP	UNCOOKED	COOKED
Cream of wheat	2 level tablespoons	½ cup
Dried beans	3 tablespoons	⅓ cup
Dried peas	3 tablespoons	⅓ cup
Grits	3 level tablespoons	½ cup
Lentils	2 tablespoons	⅓ cup
Macaroni	¼ cup	½ cup
Noodles	⅓ cup	½ cup
Oatmeal	3 level tablespoons	½ cup
Rice	2 level tablespoons	⅓ cup
Spaghetti	¼ cup	½ cup
MEAT GROUP	UNCOOKED	COOKED
Chicken	1 small drumstick	1 ounce
Chicken	½ chicken breast	3 ounces
Hamburger	4 ounces	3 ounces

APPENDIX C

Additional Resources

AMERICAN ASSOCIATION OF CLINICAL ENDOCRINOLOGISTS (AACE)
Professional organization specializing in endocrinology and high-quality patient care. Provides publications and guidelines for physicians and patient information.
www.aace.com

AMERICAN CANCER SOCIETY
Provides information on many types of cancer, including thyroid cancer.
www.cancer.org

AMERICAN THYROID ASSOCIATION
Link for a free subscription to a monthly online publication called "Clinical Thyroidology."
www.thyroid.org

ENDOCRINE AND METABOLIC DISEASES INFORMATION SERVICE
Part of the National Endocrine and Metabolic Disease Information Service. Provides brochures to the public on Graves' Disease, Hashimoto's Disease, Hyperthyroidism, Hypothyroidism, Pregnancy and Thyroid Disease, and Thyroid Function Tests.
www.endocrine.niddk.nih.gov

THE HORMONE FOUNDATION
A public resource of the Endocrine Society, this site provides outreach and education for hormone-related conditions.
www.hormone.org

LIGHT OF LIFE FOUNDATION FOR THYROID CANCER

Provides education for thyroid cancer patients and the medical community.
www.checkyourneck.com

NATIONAL CANCER INSTITUTE

Supports a national network of cancer centers and collects and distributes information on cancer research and clinical trials.
www.cancer.gov

NATIONAL GRAVES' DISEASE FOUNDATION

Supports research to find the cause and cure of Grave's Disease; provides informational publications and reports on current research
www.ngdf.org

THYROID CANCER SURVIVORS' ASSOCIATION, INC.

Provides low-iodine guidelines and cookbook, along with newsletters and a new patient packet.
www.thyca.org/rai.htm

THYROID FOUNDATION OF CANADA

Canada's national awareness program to improve the diagnosis and treatment of thyroid disease.
www.thyroid.ca

Thyroid Medication Websites

CYTOMEL (LIOTHYRONINE SODIUM) AND TAPAZOLE (METHIMAZOLE)

www.kingpharm.com

LEVOTHROID (LEVOTHYROXINE SODIUM)

www.levothroid.com

LEVOXYL (LEVOTHYROXINE SODIUM)
www.levoxyl.com

NATURE-THROID (LIOTHYRONINE AND LEVOTHYROXINE)
www.nature-throid.com

SYNTHROID (LEVOTHYROXINE SODIUM)
www.synthroid.com

THYROGEN (TSH, USED IN THYROID CANCER PATIENTS FOR DIAGNOSTICS)
www.genzyme.com

THYROLAR (TRIIODOTHYRONINE AND LEVOTHYROXINE SODIUM)
www.thyrolar.com

UNITHROID (LEVOTHYROXINE SODIUM)
www.unithroid.com

WESTHROID (LIOTHYRONINE AND LEVOTHYROXINE)
www.wes-throid.com

Standard U.S./Metric Measurement Conversions

VOLUME CONVERSIONS

U.S. Volume Measure	Metric Equivalent
⅛ teaspoon	0.5 milliliters
¼ teaspoon	1 milliliters
½ teaspoon	2 milliliters
1 teaspoon	5 milliliters
½ tablespoon	7 milliliters
1 tablespoon (3 teaspoons)	15 milliliters
2 tablespoons (1 fluid ounce)	30 milliliters
¼ cup (4 tablespoons)	60 milliliters
⅓ cup	90 milliliters
½ cup (4 fluid ounces)	125 milliliters
⅔ cup	160 milliliters
¾ cup (6 fluid ounces)	180 milliliters
1 cup (16 tablespoons)	250 milliliters
1 pint (2 cups)	500 milliliters
1 quart (4 cups)	1 liter (about)

WEIGHT CONVERSIONS

U.S. Weight Measure	Metric Equivalent
½ ounce	15 grams
1 ounce	30 grams
2 ounces	60 grams
3 ounces	85 grams
¼ pound (4 ounces)	115 grams
½ pound (8 ounces)	225 grams
¾ pound (12 ounces)	340 grams
1 pound (16 ounces)	454 grams

OVEN TEMPERATURE CONVERSIONS

Degrees Fahrenheit	Degrees Celsius
200 degrees F	100 degrees C
250 degrees F	120 degrees C
275 degrees F	140 degrees C
300 degrees F	150 degrees C
325 degrees F	160 degrees C
350 degrees F	180 degrees C
375 degrees F	190 degrees C
400 degrees F	200 degrees C
425 degrees F	220 degrees C
450 degrees F	230 degrees C

BAKING PAN SIZES

American	Metric
8 x 1½ inch round baking pan	20 x 4 cm cake tin
9 x 1½ inch round baking pan	23 x 3.5 cm cake tin
1 x 7 x 1½ inch baking pan	28 x 18 x 4 cm baking tin
13 x 9 x 2 inch baking pan	30 x 20 x 5 cm baking tin
2 quart rectangular baking dish	30 x 20 x 3 cm baking tin
15 x 10 x 2 inch baking pan	30 x 25 x 2 cm baking tin (Swiss roll tin)
9 inch pie plate	22 x 4 or 23 x 4 cm pie plate
7 or 8 inch Springform pan	18 or 20 cm Springform or loose bottom cake tin
9 x 5 x 3 inch loaf pan	23 x 13 x 7 cm or 2 lb narrow loaf or pate tin
1½ quart casserole	1.5 litre casserole
2 quart casserole	2 litre casserole

Index

We Have EVERYTHING® on Anything!

With more than 19 million copies sold, the Everything® series has become one of America's favorite resources for solving problems, learning new skills, and organizing lives. Our brand is not only recognizable—it's also welcomed.

The series is a hand-in-hand partner for people who are ready to tackle new subjects—like you!

For more information on the Everything® series, please visit *www.adamsmedia.com*

The Everything® list spans a wide range of subjects, with more than 500 titles covering 25 different categories:

Business	History	Reference
Careers	Home Improvement	Religion
Children's Storybooks	Everything Kids	Self-Help
Computers	Languages	Sports & Fitness
Cooking	Music	Travel
Crafts and Hobbies	New Age	Wedding
Education/Schools	Parenting	Writing
Games and Puzzles	Personal Finance	
Health	Pets	